"In *Somatic Practice in Yoga Therapy* Jaime has synthesized for you her decades of practice and teaching of yoga therapy with her equal depth of study in major somatic approaches to healing. If you are interested in attaining more ease, knowledge, skill, and insight in your yoga practice and in guiding others with dynamic clarity, this is the book you have been searching for. It exists!"

—Bonnie Bainbridge Cohen, Developer of Body-Mind Centering®

"If you practice yoga in any form, especially if you share it as a healing modality, *Somatic Practice in Yoga Therapy* will be an indispensable resource for work with self and others on the journey. Dr. Schmitt is masterful at integrating multiple streams of wisdom into practical tools; such a gift!"

—Carrie Demers M.D., Medical Director of PureRejuv Wellness Center, Himalayan Institute

"Novel and innovative, Dr. Schmitt has written an elegant experiential manual for those that want to feel closer to themselves somatically, utilize the body to move into deeper states of being, and encounter their own consciousness with the full force of their embodied life. A learning resource essential for students and teachers of yoga therapy and other somatic practices that will be a significant aid in the work of healing the health crises of the modern world."

—Molly McManus C-IAYT, IAYT Board President and Director
of Yoga North International SomaYoga Institute

"Steeped in history and philosophy that makes the multiplicity of yogic journeys available to anyone interested, *Somatic Practice in Yoga Therapy* unfolds as a creative journey into awareness. It has a delicious focus on deepening your bodily awareness, becoming more effective as a mover, diving into your own personal growth, and finding rich spiritual pathways to unity."

—Dr. Martha Eddy, Co-Author of *Dynamic Embodiment of the Sun Salutation*,
Director of Dynamic Embodiment Somatic Movement Therapy Training

of related interest

Somatics in Action
A Mindful and Physical Conditioning Tool for Movers
Lauren W Kearns
Forewords by Gerri Houlihan and Elizabeth Lowe Ahearn
ISBN 978 1 90914 164 3
eISBN 978 1 90914 165 0

Yoga and Somatics for Immune and Respiratory Health
Charlotte Watts
Foreword by Joanne Avison
ISBN 978 1 83997 087 0
eISBN 978 1 83997 088 7

Awakening Somatic Intelligence
Understanding, Learning and Practicing the Alexander
Technique, Feldenkrais Method and Hatha Yoga
Graeme Lynn
Foreword by Michael D. Frederick
ISBN 978 1 84819 334 5
eISBN 978 0 85701 290 6

SOMATIC PRACTICE IN YOGA THERAPY

Explorations of body, movement, mind, and self

Jaime Stover Schmitt Ed.D., C-IAYT

Foreword by Swami Rudra Ravi Bharati,
Rudolph Ballentine M.D.

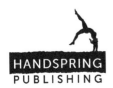

HANDSPRING
PUBLISHING

First published in Great Britain in 2024 by Handspring Publishing, an imprint of Jessica Kingsley Publishers
Part of John Murray Press

1

ISBN 978 1 91342 651 4
eISBN 978 1 91342 652 1

Printed and bound in the United States by Integrated Books International

Jessica Kingsley Publishers' policy is to use papers that are natural, renewable and recyclable
products and made from wood grown in sustainable forests. The logging and manufacturing
processes are expected to conform to the environmental regulations of the country of origin.

Handspring Publishing
Carmelite House
50 Victoria Embankment
London EC4Y 0DZ

www.handspringpublishing.com

John Murray Press
Part of Hodder & Stoughton Limited
An Hachette UK Company

Contents

Foreword

It is difficult to grasp the overwhelmingly comprehensive nature of this master work. But let's start with the context of its appearance:

The western mind is drastically split from the body. We have been bemoaning that fact for many decades. But mere intellectual discussions about the split have not done much to heal it. Yet, as Dr. Schmitt demonstrates tirelessly in her landmark book, *Somatic Practice in Yoga Therapy*, the reintegration of the mind and body can be accomplished. This is done by painstakingly and patiently knitting them back together, bit by bit, through movement, visualization, and the progressive awakening of kinesthetic awareness and the cultivation of what might be considered a sort of "somatic literacy"—as is supported by illustrations and descriptions throughout her book.

She mines the most vivid examples of such integral self-awareness from the traditional teachings of yoga, Tantra, and Ayurveda, to bring to life the quality of self-awareness that is the foundation of health, vitality, and spiritual unfoldment. This is not, however, an esoteric approach that might be in danger of languishing indefinitely in the shadows. Rather, she works from a lifetime immersion in current disciplines such as of Body-Mind Centering™, Laban Movement Analysis, and Alexander Technique, which she weaves flawlessly into her training in Indian traditions. And she does so by following the classic thread: from gross to subtle to subtler... culminating with somatic practices for self-inquiry and reflection and finally, somatic practice for union: yoga.

An example of the span of her grasp is her treatment of the vagus nerve: by bringing together what yoga has long known, and what the latest neuroscience polyvagal theory has pieced together, she demonstrates how many of our most advanced discoveries, such as the importance of the vagus nerve in the phenomenon of stress syndromes, have been present in the teachings of yoga for over a millennium.

Such magical touches, offered matter-of-factly, ultimately demonstrate the fundamental necessity of a fullness of embodiment for all true healing and transformation. We can lean again and again on Dr. Schmitt's steady hand as she repairs, reconnects, and reopens the door to a fuller, more conscious way of being on the planet...

Swami Rudra Ravi Bharati, Rudolph Ballentine M.D.

Introduction

Yoga, as is true for any authentic spiritual tradition, is about freedom rather than rigid doctrines or mere belief. It is experiential and experimental.

Georg Feuerstein (Feuerstein, 2001, para. 7, courtesy of Yoga International Inc.)

WHAT IS MODERN YOGA THERAPY?

Yoga therapy is both old and new. It would be hard to imagine that the therapeutic use of yoga for a specific concern has never been, at least in part, a faction of yoga's storyline. Certainly uncovering and working through one's impediments along the path to wholeness is the work that faces any earnest yoga practitioner, no matter at what level of being, from body to soul, the impediment appears. Yet today's repurposing and confinement of yoga to a healing modality—multi-level and holographic though it may be—has a more medical leaning. It tends to involve modifying and applying what are understood to be yoga principles and practices to special, usually health-related, needs. The knowledge base necessary to do so safely and effectively has been corralled into sets of standards and competencies by various organizations, a leader of which is the International Association of Yoga Therapists (IAYT). This worldwide professional organization accredits yoga therapist training programs and is committed to advancing yoga therapy education, training, and research, as well as to educating the public as to what yoga therapy is and what it can

do. Its mission is to establish yoga as a recognized and respected therapy (IAYT, n.d.).

One of the marvelous ways yoga serves as a therapeutic intervention is its ability to check so many of the boxes of therapeutic work. Certainly, for stress management, emotional regulation, and resilience training, its various techniques have been found to operate on multiple levels. For instance, yoga therapy can employ top–down methods or a cognitive approach that involves examining thought patterns, interactions, decisions, and strategizing solutions to life's many challenges. Through contemplative self-study and yoga meditation, practices such as these increase self-awareness and self-compassion, and promote self-acceptance and non-attachment (Demers, 2022).

Yoga techniques can also focus on a bottom-up, or body-centered, somatic approach, attending to interoceptive sensations from the body, working with grounding and breathing to directly influence the autonomic system and vagal tone. If so chosen, we can then use a blended approach to attend to and understand sensations and impressions that have come up. And we can learn to repattern our system toward less reactivity and fear. Instead, as we practice over time, we increase our capacity for self-management and self-care. By applying yoga-based adapted-for-the circumstance-and-person practices, we can build new neural circuitry in both cases. This seems to be what the yogis have been all about for centuries.

WHAT IS TRADITIONAL YOGA?

There's been recent sport in "debunking" the claim to a singular universal 5000-year-old yoga tradition, complete with a set of universally recognized yoga postures. Evidence that supports the modern yoga practices, especially those coming from south India with their great articulation of physical direction, are modern constructs influenced by western gymnastics and physical culture.

Yet yoga is generally said to have developed over a span of thousands of years. Scholars have made inroads into piecing together a narrative of yoga's past. Early research on yoga's origins carries with it a variety of Euro-Christian presumptions about what a spiritual tradition or religious practice needs to look like. Geoffrey Samuel in *The Origins of Yoga and Tantra* (2008) points to this era of research as looking for yoga through a textual elite bias that bypasses the fact that yogis of all prior eras lived mostly on the outskirts of society with practices taught through an oral tradition passed individually from teacher to student. That which was written, was done so in sutra form, which is a terse encapsulation, sort of like a shorthand that could be understood by someone already familiar with the context and culture of the statement's import. This mode of recording was for those already in the know of the broader context, principles, aims, and methodology of the practice. The culture, environment, and other specific practicalities were not captured in the texts, so when scholars worked to reconstruct yoga's early evolution, there was little evidence as to what the actual practices were, how they were to be done, on what conditions and the like. Also, what was discovered was interpreted through the lens of later frameworks, so that little reliable information remains on the actual practices of yoga from ancient times.

The Christian lens may also have predisposed researchers to look for what they knew to be religious. They could relate to an iconic leader, a "Jesus of yoga," a bible per se, and an assumption of exclusivity in the way that Protestants and Catholics don't mix. Yet mixing elements of a thread of practice seems to be more the norm throughout the long storyline of yoga than the exception. The traditional thread that I'm teaching from is considered a singular tradition made up of a combination of several distinct threads. It is a well-structured progression, meeting students at various stages of readiness and leading them through different levels of practice. It is also personalized. In this lifetime, I have veered slightly to the teachings of a faction of my tradition as they were of necessity to me. Each person is expected to follow their own inner guidance system, their *spandashakti*, as best as they are able. Personalized practice is a feature of yoga therapy as well.

A key factor in the tradition of yoga from which I teach is experience. We study scripture or literature and oral guidance, relating it to our own direct experience of the results of applying the principles through practice. Yoga practices are done to alter the experience of the individual practicing them. For instance, we perform a relaxation and breathing practice that produces an experience of our heart rate and blood pressure going down. It is a body-mind phenomenon. And, as the saying goes, "it's an inside job."

I find it interesting to note that while current yoga research looks for reliable data to debunk yoga's past and prove yoga's efficacy, there is a rise in trauma-sensitive approaches to yoga. These approaches acknowledge the value of subjective experience in the body as an important element in effective therapeutic intervention. It's no secret that the western world has valued thinking over feeling, and that the information the body registers even below our ability to cogitate on its message has not been considered relevant. Stephen Porges, author of *The Polyvagal Theory* (2011), states:

> Only during the past 50 years have emotion and investigation of subjective states of feeling become an accepted research domain within psychology. Prior research and its clinical treatment models emphasized the cognitive pathway with the objective of nurturing cognitive functions and containing subjective feelings. This focus emphasized objective, measurable indices of behaviors and cognitive functions while dismissing subjective reports of feelings. (p. 34)

So as western scholars search for the real or authentic yoga, it is important to note that they may not recognize it. And if they do, they may not value it as it does not, like the square peg of subjective experience, fit neatly into the round hole of the patriarchally based evidential science.

The traditional yoga to which I refer throughout this work is a philosophy and lifestyle passed down directly through a lineage of teachers by a primarily oral tradition. This tradition does include preparatory and associated practices that attach to a deep and far-reaching philosophical framework. The practices function as archetypes, as malleable forms that provide a menu of options for the principles they put into play. In this scenario, a skilled practitioner has used several to many of the various practices and knows them intimately. It is an intimacy born of painstaking practice and self-observation of effect over time, usually with the guidance of a more advanced practitioner or adept.

This approach to yoga in general is not much different than an orientation to yoga therapy that invites the therapist to have good experiential grounding in yoga practice. This may pertain to poses, breathing practice, meditative techniques and the like, and includes a regulated lifestyle with a basic understanding of Ayurvedic remedies and moral practices encompassed in the *yama* and *niyama*.

Yoga therapy, at least in its early form, relies heavily on the therapist-practitioner's experience with the practices of yoga. What a therapist-practitioner gives as a practice may be largely based on their experience of the effect and efficacy of such practice in their own life. In fact, a yogic adept has this as a defining feature; they master the practices of the yoga applied to themselves! This is a unique model for healthcare workers. Unlike the western model of healthcare, in which a physician need not (and should not) partake of the remedies prescribed in order to know what they do, a yoga therapist performs best when they have first-hand experience of the effects of breathing, relaxation, and mindfulness practices: the nuances of which are known only through direct experience. A surgeon does not try out the procedures on themselves. An acupuncturist may do some self-needling, and massage therapists get massages, but yogis run their own self-studies and research projects on themselves. This depth of practice allows the practitioner to better guide their clients.

The notion of being a practitioner is important here because we are talking about the doing of mental and physical techniques, not just reading about them and their benefits. Yoga is performed on oneself. The therapist is not doing a yogic treatment, but teaching, guiding, and relating to the client from the standpoint of the yogic frame of reference.

Benefit comes from doing the practice, not from knowledge of the practice. The benefit can be registered through data collected physically, like the lowering of blood pressure or weight loss. But it may also register within that individual's experience. The yoga therapy client may feel better, have less fear and more hope. They may gradually become less reactive and more understanding of others' points of view. It is difficult to isolate individual causal relationships—"I did 30 minutes of practice, so that meant I only yelled twice at my kids today"—yet the transformational aspects of patient practice over time can be profound.

From this perspective, then, I'm considering traditional yoga to be an orientation to life for which its adepts have developed a host of practices based on principles articulating a philosophical point of view that entails mental and physical cultivation aimed at insight and liberation. This philosophy, with the principles that articulate it along with adaptable methods of practice, has been passed down through the generations of practitioners.

The fact that there are teachers alive today who hold parts, or all, of a lineage's teachings makes a yoga tradition a living one. Samaya Sri Vidya Tantra was brought to the United States in 1969 by Sr. Swami Rama of the Himalayas. He founded the Himalayan Institute, headquartered in northeastern Pennsylvania since 1977. He taught students at many levels of entry. One of his early main students branched to a specialization. And this is how it seems to go with modern-day yoga clans. The teachings remain infused with the traditional thread yet are adapted and applied to varying needs and populations. I've had the extreme good fortune to be a student of H. H. Sri Swami Rama, and his protégé, Pandit Rajmani Tigunait Ph.D., along with two of his early main disciples, if I may use that term liberally, Dr. Rudolph Ballentine M.D., now Swami Rudra Ravi, and Dr. Joan Shivarpita Harrigan. Ballentine has distilled and modernized several principles of Tantra, teaching out of his ashram in North Carolina. Harrigan met H. H. Sri Swami Chadrasekharan and, the lineage *acharya* of a specialized offshoot. This branch of yoga focuses on more subtle work with individuals who are ready for it, called Kundalini Vidya.

TANTRA AS AN EMBODIED PATH

Even when a tradition is cited, as I am attempting to do here, it is important to remember that a non-western view of multiplicity and complexity organized by a vision or underlying purpose is at play. This is because the traditional yoga brought to the United States by Swami Rama consists of tiered elements of Patanjali Yoga, Advaita Vedanta, and Sri Vidya Tantra. Working systematically through practices from each of these approaches allows the teacher of this work to meet a variety of students where they are in their development and to progress them accordingly along a path of insight and refinement. Generally this tradition is called the tradition of the Himalayan Masters and Samaya Sri Vidya Tantra.

Tantra in the west is often misunderstood. So here is an extremely brief orientation to where this approach is placed. There are three main versions of Tantra: Kaula, which is the one most known in the west, Samaya, which is the path described in this book, and Mishra, which indicates a mixture of the other two.

If you've heard of Tantra, you've likely heard of left-handed or right-handed Tantra. These two distinctions are both part of Kaula Tantra, which focuses on enacting rituals. Because this requires actions it is called external. Left-handed Tantrics may even use intoxicants, mudras, and sexual contact. The right-handed Tantrics perform these rituals only symbolically.

The Samaya school of Tantra is a practice without external rituals. Its purpose is liberation. Swami Jhaneshvara Bharati, a teacher of the tradition, says Samaya means "I am with you" (n.d., Samaya Tantra section, para. 2). This is a reference to an indwelling force beneath and before the life force of prana, called Shakti. Shakti is one side of the coin of the duality of existence, Shiva being the other. Shakti is the motive force. Through practice this divine inner companion within each individual, called Kundalini Shakti, is activated and moves toward spiritual union. Three features of what I have understood from my time with these teachers and my own practice stand out as pointedly relevant to somatic practice in yoga therapy. They are that all of nature is seen as Tantra's toolbox, everything is everything, and everything is an experiment.

Nature is Tantra's toolbox

As a westerner, I was brought up to think of myself as an individual, an entity alone in a world in which I would need to find my way. The practice of yoga I was taught brought me into relationship with a deeper identity, one in which I experienced myself as part of a great whole. As I studied the path of healing through this tradition, I was made aware of the premise in Tantra, that nature, including human nature, the laws of physics, and the properties operating the natural world was the natural tool of yoga. Yoga was a framework, not just a list of poses, and not just a culture-bound Indian ideology. It was truly, as Swami Rama and others taught, a systematic science of self-transformation, and nature was its toolbox. The codified practices of body, breath, mental focus, diet, relaxation, and balanced living were operational strategies that worked because they were grounded in, and worked closely with, the laws of nature, the laws of physics, and of biological life.

This meant that as a practitioner with proper guidance and diligent practice became increasingly adept they could also modify and devise variations on these themes for the sake of personal evolution. And this was because nature and all that it entails is at the disposal of a yogic adept from this tradition.

I use nature here to mean that which we know to be the real world, with all the laws and properties discoverable through research and experimentation. Tantra, of which I speak, positions us as part of and also as above this world. As Alan Watts (n.d.) remarked, "You are something that the whole universe is doing in the same way that a wave is something that the whole ocean is doing." So to experience ourselves individually we also experience nature collectively. This tradition of yoga uses natural principles and features of the natural world as a fulcrum to move us on the path of evolution. As we study ourselves by paying close attention to our tendencies proficiencies, our movement patterns and ways of using our bodies, what works for us in terms of food choices, energy management, kinds of practices, and all the rest, we are studying our own corporeal nature. As we learn more about the nature of ourselves in relation to our world, we begin to understand who we are.

Everything is everything

There is a saying from the Puranas, "*yat pinde tat brahmande*," the universe is (in) the body and the body is (in) the universe, or whatever is in the microcosm is also in the macrocosm. This widespread ancient view is holographic, and a good guide for work in the context of yoga therapy. In *Radical Healing: Integrating the World's Great Therapeutic Traditions to Create a New Transformative Medicine* (1999, p. 5) Rudolph Ballentine writes, "From a holistic perspective, our suffering comes from forgetting our wholeness. The word health comes from the Anglo Saxon *häl* whence also come *heal* and *whole*. Perhaps the simplest definition of *healing* is 'to make whole'". This whole includes a dimension of that which lies beyond the body and the mind, from a yogic point of view. The knowing of that beyond is an experience beyond experience. There is a point at which it is not an academic pursuit. The point of departure to union is an experiential one.

Yoga therapists lean heavily on a similar yogic model that articulates five progressively subtler bodies that are seen to comprise our personality. Described in the Taittiriya Upanishad, these five bodies, called *koshas*, or "sheaths" in Sanskrit, are imaged as fitting one inside the next like concentric rings. Only the outermost and densest layer consists of physical matter. The four internal ones are subtle and invisible to most methods of physical data gathering. They can be sensed somatically and subjectively by us when we pay close attention. Some yoga practices are designed to train the practitioner to sense and work with these deeper levels of being. And because yoga holds that these inner layers of being are more potently influential in our health, and also that the deepest levels move with us through many lifetimes, yogis focused on practices to refine and purify each of these levels specifically.

The good news is that working at one level affects other levels as well. So we don't need our clients to be adept yogis to see gains in wellness and self-understanding. This model and this holographic point of view allows us to leverage one area of being from another, and can be a very useful principle in helping clients progress along their trajectory to wholeness.

Everything is an experiment

My teachers were all "yoga scientists" in that they taught us to run the experiments of yoga practice. Looking for better digestion? Change your diet. What did that do? Stimulate your *agni* (digestive fire). What was the result? Now process your emotions. What results did you get? They instructed us to not necessarily believe we would get the results promised, but to run the experiment by doing the practice and checking in internally to sense the result.

This approach takes the practice of yoga out of the realm of sanctimonious commandment to one of playful investigation. In *Radical Healing* (1999) Rudolph Ballentine goes so far as to invite this exploratory attitude in the face of difficult medical diagnoses. Rather than meeting the diagnosis with fear and helplessness, he suggests becoming curious about how this situation has come into being. And then get to the work of transformation of self the symptoms are calling for. A radical move, but one that arises out of the Tantric model of doing your own self-research.

These experiments require tuning in and paying attention to our own embodied experience. What sensation do we notice within our body? What tissues seem to be involved? What emotions and level of inward or outward focus do they engender? Do we feel safe and secure, or do we feel on alert for danger? Is there a sense of connection with something greater than our own ego-identity?

As yoga therapy evolves into a more readily accepted healthcare modality, my hope is that innovative methods of validation for these interoceptive and neuroceptive states evolve, like Stephen Porges' polyvagal theory. Through the creative applications of yoga's traditional practices, patients and clients can find their way toward a new paradigm of healing that includes personal transformation.

WHAT ARE SOMATIC PRACTICES?

Somatic practices are things we do that bring us into an experience of ourselves through our body. You might ask: how else can we know ourselves to be? In our head is one answer. Shutting down and not paying attention to the body's many cries for movement, for a change of position, or for even a drink of water is another.

In 1976 philosophy professor and movement

therapist Thomas Hanna coined the term "somatics" to indicate a collective work that involved self-reference through the body. Common features of various types of somatic practice were body knowledge and awareness focused on internal sensing and perception, movement analysis and awareness, and hands-on practices that involved the felt sense or lived experience of the "soma" or body in Greek. In Hanna's words, "Somatics is the study of the self from the perspective of one's lived experience, encompassing the dimensions of body, psyche, and spirit" (Hanna, n.d., para. 2).

A host of body-mind techniques and methods of exploration and inquiry fall into this field, from early modern dance trailblazers who moved from within rather than from a performance perspective, to individuals seeking to improve vocal or physical performance, to those seeking new inventive modes of authentic expression during performance.

So, a somatic practice is something you engage in that brings you into greater awareness of your experience of your body: how it feels, how it's doing, how it moves, what it consists of, and what comes up for you as you tune in.

If self-referencing through the body is key in somatic practice, then yoga may well be the mother of all somatic practices. The fact that much of the modern, as well as ancient, somatic work is showing up in both physical and mental therapeutic contexts is evidence that the felt experience of the body is crucial to our understanding of self and our ability to find a level of comfort, strength and connection necessary to face life as it is in our world today.

How to Use this Book

This book falls in pedagogical line with the ways I was taught as a student of the embodied practice of yoga. There is explanation and, at times, discussion, and then practice and reflection. I've tried to give a broad view of the ways in which I've employed somatic practice in my private and group yoga therapy for over three decades, and in our training and continuing education programs. In a book such as this I only have room to give you a set of examples of how this goes and can go. My hope is that you'll use these somatizations and explorations as points of departure for further self-research and study. They are openings to exploration and this collection is nowhere near exhaustive. I encourage you to follow your physical instincts and your deeper intuitions. None of this is offered as finite or pat, but as discoveries of avenues to ongoing investigation into the mystery of which we all are the embodiment.

Because this is a journey of exploration, I invite you to approach the practices or somatizations in this book with self-awareness and agency. Please engage in a way that is comfortable to you. I encourage you to only do what you want and, if you like, check in with yourself, and your responses to the work as you explore. I ask also that you pay attention to how you feel and what comes up for you as you try things out. Here are some other possible ideas you may wish to consider as you work with your own embodiment in this book and beyond it.

Please consider:

- enacting your own inner witness, like you would establish in meditation
- giving yourself enough time to practice, and have some time open afterwards as well
- having what I call a tether, someone around not doing the exploring at the same time you're exploring and that you can reach out to if you like
- exploring in an open clear space in which you won't be disturbed and from which you have a clear exit
- reminding yourself you can stop at any point. If you wish to stop at a certain time, set a timer and honor yourself by stopping when you said you would
- reading the step-by-step instructions first
- perhaps exploring with one or more people
- when you complete a practice, taking some time to draw, write, journal, move or process in any way that suits you if you like.

This book will address somatic practices in yoga therapy in four main ways. We'll explore somatic practices for body understanding, movement efficiency, self-inquiry and as the path of yoga's goal of union.

First we'll explore how embodying anatomical location and physiological function can give insight and command in observation and remedial practice. A challenge for students of yoga therapy is not only the somewhat daunting task of gaining a good grasp of anatomy and physiology, but to discern what of this voluminous content will be truly useful and relevant to their client practice. Beyond this quest for delimitation is the translation process of getting the terminology and images off the pages and into an applicable use aimed at clients' bodies. The first section thus focuses on learning methods that do just that—take anatomy off the page and into experience.

The second section is focused on improving movement efficiency, which in my experience as a yoga therapist is a big part of how we can help our clients. Pain reduction and energy conservation are often welcome benefits of better bodily use. Learning to move better is a process that requires attention and relearning. How does attending to our own bodily awareness improve our ability to move well through our lives? What are ways to affect this in someone else? Rather than present a singular system of body reorganization through somatic practice, here I'll lay out fundamental features of improved movement efficiency. When these foundational understandings are in place, any number of combinations of approaches can then be developed and shared from them. They are also fun to explore!

The next section deals with the body as a vehicle of self-understanding with movement as the medium of its expression. What does the body reveal? What might symptoms be trying to say? What are the messages coming through our felt experience that we may want to attend to with the light of our conscious awareness? This third section explores somatic practices focused on this manner of embodied self-inquiry, which I call SRI: Self-Reflective Inquiry™. And if yoga's ancient goal is desired or in sight, no matter. This work can be of vital importance in bringing what is within into the light of awareness.

In the fourth and final section we'll come full circle returning to traditional yoga and its ancient goal of self-liberation. As Joseph Campbell says in his interview with Bill Moyers, "the labyrinth is thoroughly known" (Moyers, 1988, para. 1). Here, we'll be reminded of the path of yoga as a solid entry onto "the royal path," a veritable yellow brick road, to the direct experience of its goal.

Section I

SOMATIC PRACTICE FOR AN EMBODIED UNDERSTANDING OF THE BODY

I hear and I forget.
I see and I remember.
I do and I understand.

Attributed to Dr. Maria Montessori (Peabody Montessori, n.d.)

INTRODUCTION: HOW TO USE THESE PRACTICES

On the value of embodied learning for yoga therapy

The amount of anatomical learning that can be acquired in the pursuit of competency in an emerging healthcare field can be overwhelming, especially for those who do not come from a foundation with anatomy as its center. Even if one learns the anatomical names, movements, positions, and locations, this learning does not automatically translate into clinical practice. And it is this translation process that is so necessary to the acquisition of practical skill in observation, analysis, and treatment delivery.

This is one reason why embodied understanding of the body can be important to the yoga therapist. It focuses the learning on the familiar use of the body in posture and in motion. This is as true for "mere mortals" in everyday bodily

use as it is for professional athletes and other performers. It is also an extremely helpful way to develop command of the understanding of the body in the effort to help teachers and practitioners of yoga, dance, martial arts, massage, and other physical practices improve their movement and physical skill in action.

In my experience as a yoga therapist I am far better able to "see" into my clients' bodies when I have myself spent time locating the involved structures, tissues, and processes in my own body, and then in others'. This is because I'm not only hoping to understand location but also function. How do these various tissues and parts work together? How is this person (sometimes this person is me!) using their body and is that working well for them? If there is pain, joint wearing, tissue damage, or the like, I'm seeking to understand what is awry as specifically and inclusively as possible. It is from this baseline of observation that I can then set to the steady work of unravelling the history of those tissues with the goal to repattern into wholeness and fuller, easeful use.

As a somatic practitioner I need to be able to, at some point in the process, envision. I need to get a whole picture of what is happening in the tissues and in the functioning of the body area so that I can then see what need to be the steps to take in rehabilitation.

TO MORE FULLY COMPREHEND THE FELT EXPERIENCE

The story of what unfolds as I follow the path of crumbs is the evidence in the body's tissues. It may not rest solely in the physical properties, weights and levers, wear and tear of joints and tissues of the body. The body's story may, and often does, reveal deeper reasons for movement choices and features of alignment. It may be that a woman who rounds her shoulders forward and drops her chest was harassed and embarrassed by her growing breasts in middle school and carried this body posture into her adult way of being in her world. It may be that the story of low back pain of a man in his fifties unfolds a deep and pervasive fear of not having enough money, time, love, freedom, energy to meet the growing demands in his family, his work life, and his soul's desires.

To take this one step further, to a large degree the process of conceptualization is based in our body. Our bodily experience is our preverbal baseline orientation, our starting point for understanding ourselves.

We interact with our environment through movement. In utero we move in amniotic fluid and experience our body's form and substance in relation to the growing firmness of the uterine wall. As we continue to grow, we sense the downward pull of gravity. During our first year, we struggle to organize and gain control over our body to move towards what we want and away from what we don't. We experience gravity giving us the direction of down as a felt phenomenon. From there, other-than-down becomes our matrix of spatial awareness that, as we organize

our movement capability, we move into and through.

All this happens in the context of our sense of safety in relation to our environment, which includes others and objects in the world around us. Are we able to bond to the earth or our mother's embrace, or do we withdraw, hold ourselves away, not merging or yielding our body's weight? Do we find ourselves defending before we even know what is happening? How do we do that and what is the result? How do we find comfort and support? How successfully are we able to exert our will to have our needs met and our curiosity satisfied? And are we able to find ways to withdraw into ourselves for rest and renewal?

These early rhythms of going out and coming in, as we refine our orientation to the environment of gravity and space, and the subsequent solutions we find through movement for doing so, lay down the pathways for our later development. How we organize ourselves is a felt phenomenon; it is lived and relived through the experience of our body and its movement solutions in gravity through space. Yoga is the practice of becoming aware of our patterns of orientation and action. Stephen Porges (2011) writes about the early development of the autonomic nervous system as providing the neural platform for social behavior, as his focus is on articulating various aspects of how our autonomic system helps us survive. Our early development sets up the template for our interactions. Our individual manner of asserting and withdrawing, opening and closing, going toward or away, gathering and scattering, and all manner of polar rhythmic change rely on this foundation. Yoga practice brings us into an aware exploration, a multi-level reexamination, of our manner of being in the world, including our ability to ride this continuum of autonomic regulation.

Our lived experience of our body's movement in space, how we organize ourselves in daily life, gives us the ground for abstraction. We make meaning from our embodied experience of self in our world. Physical space, sensation, and movement are the ways we know our selves to be and form the foundation for later learning.

We can learn to attend to, feel, and be present to what is happening and how our body and its autonomic system participates. Or we can ignore, cover up with other patterns, and not take the time to allow these deeper processes to come into awareness. Yoga practice can be a way to open ourselves to these subtle, yet physical ways of relating to ourselves and our environment. This is at the heart of somatic work, of which yoga is one systematic approach.

TO LEARN ANATOMY AND PHYSIOLOGY THROUGH SOMATIC PRACTICE

Taking anatomy, or what I think of as the geography of the body, off the page or screen of two dimensions and into lived experience becomes the basis of an informed practice that mimics the somatic wisdom of the yogic adepts. Learning anatomy, anatomical concepts, kinesiology, and movement analysis in an experiential way gives the learner the ability to translate the knowledge into practice more readily. If I know the location and action of a muscle as I move, I can better see it on someone else. I feel the scaffolding and support of my own bones to sense and imagine what my client's body structure feels like to them and how their body "handles" in movement. The support my organs give to the volume of my torso, and to my sense of ease and comfort, will be a baseline for comparison, as I observe, examine and interview the person before explaining their digestive issues and sense of dis-ease.

The sky's the limit when it comes to ways to learn about the body somatically. You may think at first that some of these seem like child's play. But that simplicity of experience has purpose. Playful exploration is highly valued in experiential learning. Safe and enjoyable exploration opens us to new possibilities and that is often what is needed in the quest for healing beyond the naming of diagnosis.

WAYS OF TEACHING SOMATIC PRACTICES TO LEARN ABOUT THE BODY

Learning about the body's anatomy and physiology is often in the context of medical practice, in which students must memorize a large number of facts in short amounts of time. Among other things this serves the function of ensuring that providers have the proper background for their clinical practice to communicate effectively with common terminology. While this is also important to the practice of yoga therapy, the experience of the patient or client in practice is of tantamount importance. Guiding individuals in checking in with themselves and their bodies is a large part of realizing the efficacy of yoga practice and of the sometimes incremental changes that take place when applied in a therapeutic role. How are they feeling before and after the practices? Has their pain level decreased? Are they less fearful, fatigued, stiff, or sore? Can they move better? Can they do more of what they want to do?

The constituent elements of somatic study and practices listed below sometimes get lumped together under the heading of intuition. I want to leave a space for this untrackable instantaneous experience of perception. Other times, the realization or download of sensory information may simply be so fast that we're not able to grasp how an impression or insight came. We each have our own way of best orienting to new ideas, new information, and new approaches to understanding and integrating what we learn. Some areas of exploration will be more comfortable and familiar, others less so. Each has its own advantages and disadvantages.

The areas for somatically based learning about the body can be combined in multifarious ways! For the sake of outlining our approach, main areas are listed with the hope that in practice you'll mix them with one another according to your curiosity and purpose. In practice you may begin with one and be drawn into other areas that would yield different ways of perceiving, or you may simply find yourself transitioning from one to others as you follow your interest and play with what you uncover. The various modes of perception we use in our teaching, client session preparation, study, and work with clients are listed below, with some non-exhaustive ideas for how you might explore.

Visual

Visual images are an excellent resource for learning anatomy and physiology. It's good to have several versions of the same image. Drawings and paintings done by a human being have gone through that person's understanding and expression. I find these to be exceptionally valuable because of that. Computer-generated images can be helpful in a different way, especially as many can be rotated so you see the topic in question from various angles and points of view. The *Netter Atlas of Human Anatomy* (Netter, 2022) is the bible of anatomical plates and is worth looking for. It is often available used or secondhand. If you're okay with them, images from anatomical dissection can be useful as well, especially when anomalies are important.

Visual images and observation

The ways we use visual images in our teaching, client session preparation, study, and work with clients concerning anatomy and physiology are as follows:

- *Still images*: The use of still anatomical images is very common. They provide an anchoring impression of the anatomical item.
- *Still images of schemata*: These can show functionality, like the lines of pull of muscles or features of anatomy superimposed over the outside of the body to show location.
- *Video images*: Sometimes videos are narrated with descriptions that highlight anatomical features.
- *Observation of an individual*: This involves looking at a person and observing what may be visible, such as bony landmarks or general location of the anatomy in question based on description and proportions. Observing several people with different proportions while locating the heart, the span of the lungs, or the endocrine glands can be a useful learning experience. This could be practiced with musculoskeletal tissues as well, such as estimating the expanse of a ligament from one bony protuberance to another, such as the lateral collateral ligament of the knee.
- *Observation of an individual in movement*: This involves gaining an impression of how well a tissue or body area functions locally and globally in the matrix of an individual's movement efficiency.

Visualizing

The ways we use visualizing in our teaching, client session preparation, study, and work with clients concerning anatomy and physiology are as follows:

- Visualization of an anatomical feature, the parts of the body participating optimally in movement, and actual physiological processes.
- Visualization as a superimposition of some feature of anatomy while observing another person (or oneself as possible). This is like a visualized overlay onto the person. This can be very helpful in repatterning movement pathways.
- Visualization of an object or action that supports correct alignment and optimal use of a body part, area, or the entire body. For instance, I can visualize warm hands on the top of my shoulders to help me lower them when typing.
- Visualization of non-anatomical images to support body use, energy flow, or liveliness of cells, or other content. I can imagine a lovely large balloon hooked onto the top of my head to allow my head to float forward and up for good sitting alignment.

Auditory

The ways we use the auditory channel of perception in our teaching, client session preparation, study, and work with clients concerning anatomy and physiology are as follows:

- Description of anatomy and physiological processes. These can be useful to get bearings and to follow along while inner sensing.
- Somatization. Guided directions to explore within the body at times using visualization, movement, and more.

Touch

The ways we use touch in our teaching, client session preparation, study, and work with clients concerning anatomy and physiology are as follows:

- Touch of self and others to feel anatomical structures through the sense of touch. This can be palpation of the bony landmarks, shapes of bones, movement of muscles under the skin, and joint movement. Here the focus mainly is on location and proportion of various anatomical features.
- Touch to image into the body. This way of touching brings us beyond simply location and into curiosity about how the tissue or bodily process is functioning. It includes touching while thinking specifically of an organ or of a function such as digestion.
- Touch as a search within the body. This is a sort of sonar of the mind. For our purpose in this section, the inquiry is kept to the realm of anatomy and physiological processes. Here, through the sense of touch, I'm looking for the tissue or function in question and searching for feedback that matches (or notably does not match) my ideation. This can also be an open question of sensing into the body and waiting for what presents itself on the screen of mind. It may be that information beyond anatomical description comes—such as an emotion, or some sort of intuitive impression that jumps the fence of one or more sensory signals, going straight to the mind through a sort of ultra-perception. This can happen for both the therapist and the client, and at times both participants have a similar experience.

Inner sensing

By inner sensing I mean whatever can be picked up by paying attention to what and how one feels in the body. This would include proprioception, which is sensing your orientation in space and your movement through mechanisms in the tissues that measure force and positioning in stillness and movement. It also includes interoception, a more contemporary term that refers to an inclusive read of the body's tissues, giving a sense of not only where and how you're moving, but how you're doing as well. It includes sensation from the viscera—the heart, lungs, and digestive tract as well as the other organs—and what registers about our state of being in any one moment.

The ways we use inner sensing in our teaching, client session preparation, study, and work with clients concerning anatomy and physiology are as follows:

- Inner sensing of the body's anatomy. We search for it, usually by having an image and/or a description which may include location, size, special features, and perhaps function.
- Inner sensing of the body's physiological processes. We reach with our awareness for these as well. This is through imagination in combination with inner sensing. I think of it as a training in perception of subtle awareness. Being around yoginis I've observed them to be extraordinarily sensitive and perceptive individuals. Rather than judge this as some sort of weakness I consider it an innate talent that can be developed toward a high level of perception in therapeutic work. From inner sensing, seeing and feeling and other avenues of awareness may be added.
- Inner sensing of emotions or mood. Even though we are keeping these avenues for exploration to the physical level of anatomy and physiology, mood

and emotion often arise as a response to the tissues being explored. While not our initial intention, we also don't wish to negate an organic felt response. So, allowing for how the client is feeling today, an association made is often useful and can be explored later in the work as deemed helpful to the client. For instance, when sensing their head a client may sense their head feels full and heavy. They feel groggy and sad. The experience of their body may not be separated from their state of emotion at the moment of their inquiry. Or someone might state, "I just noticed that when I feel my bladder, I also feel scared." While these experiences are tethered to the anatomy and physiological function of the body, the information that arises brings us into aspects of self beyond the physical. Somatic practice concerning these levels of being, such as the energetic and mental–emotional and beyond, are explored later. For now, I feel it is important not to inhibit what comes up. Yet it is also important to create a safe container for that level of work and exploration.

External sensing

This refers to all the information coming to us from what is outside of ourselves. The ways we use external sensing in our teaching, client session preparation, study, and work with clients concerning anatomy and physiology are specifically as follows:

- To locate in space beyond our body boundary. This relates to knowing where our body ends. It also helps us learn to explore the space another person inhabits with their body. If I can imagine and sense—which I do as one act, even though I need to use two words to say it—the location of a known object in space, such as where the doorknob is in my house, I can do this within another's form as well. I can sense where something is in space that I am not. It is a perceptual skill I can develop.

- To sense proximity. Proximity is how close things are to one another. Just like when you are aiming a balled-up piece of paper headed for the trash bin, you gain a sense of where your target is in space. You sense the amount of space between your projectile and the basket. Just as an artist will sense the right proportion of objects to be pictured in the painting she is painting, we sense spatially how close or far to place things in our externalized representations of our inner world. This is a relevant skill in perceiving anatomical features in another body.

Movement

The ways we use movement in our teaching, client session preparation, study, and work with clients concerning anatomy and physiology are as follows:

- Move freely and be open, like a blank slate, to what you sense and experience in each moment.
- Move to explore the body's anatomy in relation to the concepts being taught or utilized and analyzed, while focused on sensing the body part, area, or function in question.
- Move to feel an anatomical feature or kinesiological property range of motion, such as the sensing of end feel at a joint.
- Move to integrate an anatomical or physiological concept.
- Move to repattern a refined action, based on a new insight into use.

Manipulation

By manipulation I mean to do something with the hands and body, to manipulate objects somehow. This may include demonstrating the use of the body when using a tool or playing an instrument or typing at a laptop. It also refers to manipulating an object with the entire body, such as in picking up a box from squatting to standing, or other actions in which we not only touch but move and interact with things and people in our environment. We may do this to observe self and others.

Drawing

The ways we use drawing in our teaching, client session preparation, study, and work with clients concerning anatomy and physiology are as follows:

- To replicate as best we can an anatomical image, a very rewarding endeavor for understanding a specific part or area.
- To make a diagram of a physiological process.
- To draw our own experience of either or both of the above.
- To draw our impression, our sense of what our own or another person's body is doing in terms of movement, energy, emotional impression, issue, or problem.
- To have an external way to look at how we embody a particular area or part. My drawing of my own rib cage will tell me something about the way I sense it.

Modeling

The ways we use modeling in our teaching, client session preparation, study, and work with clients concerning anatomy and physiology are as follows:

- To model anatomy such as bones, organs, muscles, and really any aspect we are curious about.

- To place parts together, to build a part of the body so as to understand the parts and the way they fit and work together.
- To illustrate a process and, if people are part of what is constructed, to possibly act out the process.
- To model our experience in our body: what our felt experience is like, and then perhaps what comes up for us as we do so.

Sharing

The ways we use verbal and written sharing in our teaching, client session preparation, study, and work with clients concerning anatomy and physiology are as follows:

- To teach, share, turn, tell, and write what we capture so as to reinforce the learning and check for gaps in it, and to translate what we experience into some other form.
- To explore what has already been discovered to corroborate or get different views of a potentially collective experience.
- To be seen and heard.

CHAPTER 1

Somatic Practices for Understanding the Body's "Geography"

Experiencing Anatomy and Anatomical Concepts

A FRAMEWORK FOR EXPERIENCING SPACE: LABAN'S DIMENSIONS, DIRECTIONS, SPATIAL TENSIONS, AND FORMS

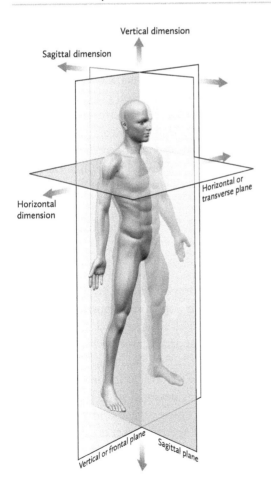

Figure 1.1 Anatomical planes

Any study of anatomy is going to begin with the anatomical planes that orient the body and its parts in space. Usually, a human figure is pictured on a page standing in the anatomical position, feet flat, legs parallel, eyes ahead, facing forward with arms at the sides, palms forward. Images of the three cardinal planes (and possibly a few minor ones) are superimposed and named (Figure 1.1). These terms become part of the language of location of the geography of the body.

This is a necessary starting point, especially for positioning a diagnostic imaging device or when cutting into live tissue. But what about the lived sense of the body in space and in the space within and around? How is that known to us and what would it give us in understanding our body geography, function, and movement? How do we record and recall our experience and awareness of space in our personal life? What does our posture and movement reveal about our inner states? And what does how we feel in occupying space we inhabit mean to us personally?

The "felt sense" is just that; what you are feeling in the moment. Experiencing space in my body and movement gives me an embodied understanding of it. If I intimately experience the space my body takes up and moves through,

I can become clearer and more precise in my subsequent observation of others. The refinement of this awareness will improve my skill in designing remedial postures and movements for myself and others.

An excellent framework for somatic exploration of space is Rudolph Laban's work called Space Harmony. Rudolph Laban was a true renaissance man who worked in many fields in the early 1900s with the thread of movement theory as his baseline for investigation (Laban & Ullmann, 2011). As a profound inspiration for subsequent artists, dancers, teachers, choreographers, and movement analysts, his students and associates carried his work into many fields of application, even though much was lost during the Nazi regime. He worked to establish a literacy of dance by recording movement in various forms of notation. Throughout his life he diligently formulated notation systems that could represent every aspect of movement in written form.

Over the years his work has been encapsulated into a unit of study called Laban Movement Analysis, which has four main areas: Body, Effort, Space, and Shape. These are germinal categories for sweepingly diverse applications of movement observation and analysis. As a theoretical framework for movement observation, his work has been applied in psychology, movement therapy, health, dance, theater, art, industry, business management, and other fields. These four main categories of investigation (body, effort, space, and shape) are integral as they are always present in our lived experience of movement. Yet we may separate them out to focus on each one individually.

One way Laban investigated the use of and expressivity implicit in our way of inhabiting space was through what he called trace forms. These look like the trails of light a Dayglo™ stick makes when waved around in the dark. Like a time-lapsed photo, a trace form is the point-by-point pathway of movement in space with each point showing the last location prior to a change in direction. Laban related these "tracings in space" or spatial pathways made by the body and its parts to geometric shapes. The main ones are the cube, the tetrahedron, and the 20-sided icosahedron. He created spatial scales and chords similar in a sense to musical scales and chords. These could be scored and performed in a timeframe similar to that of written music. These were the basis of his movement choirs in which people joined together and performed the score written in terms of space and time notation.

THE KINESPHERE

A fundamental and extremely useful term in Laban's study of space is the kinesphere. It is the space reachable by any part of the body without moving off one's place, which would require taking a step or transferring weight fully onto any other body part. The kinesphere is often readily conceived of by imagining standing in a spherical bubble of empty space. Moving in one's kinesphere usually elicits postural movement that emphasizes the space around oneself, in contrast to moving through general space in which interaction and locomotion take place. Even though in yoga *asana* (posture) practice there may often be a step up or a step back with feet together or apart, along with changes of support such as sitting, standing, lying, and the like, most of the movement is done in place and thus within one's personal space or kinesphere. Keeping to one's own yoga mat in a typical yoga class session is a sort of marker of one's "place" in space, in Laban terms.

BASIC DIRECTIONS AND LEVELS FOR ORIENTING IN SPACE SOMATICALLY

Three-dimensional space involves the vertical, sagittal, and horizontal dimensions. These three dimensions exist in relation to the field of gravity. When used with reference to the body as a whole they orient the body upright in the field of gravity. They can also refer to one body region, part, or area. Orientational directional lines can be imagined passing through the body's space and are used for location as well as for alignment and in analyzing movement efficiency.

The three dimensions, vertical, sagittal, and horizontal, make up the directional cross of axes (Figure 1.2).

Each of these dimensions has two opposing directions. Vertical has upward and downward, sagittal has forward and backward, and horizontal has right and left, sometimes referred to as side across and side open (Figure 1.3). Imagine the center of this cross is at your body's center of gravity, just below your navel center.

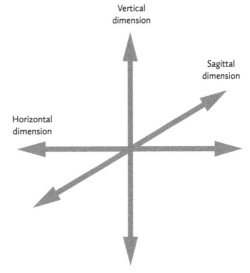

Figure 1.2 The directional cross of axes

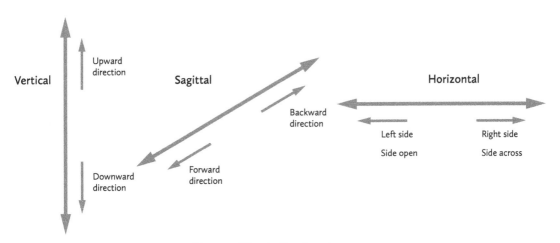

Figure 1.3 The six directions in space

From the three dimensions we get six directions. Laban devised symbols for these, as shown in Figure 1.4.

He also devised a way to notate what he termed levels of movement in space (Figure 1.5).

If you again refer to an area just below the navel as center or, as Laban will call it, place middle, movement occurring below that area will occur at a low level and movement significantly higher is at high level. Movement around the central level is middle level. He notated the levels using a dot in the center of the symbol of middle, a figure fully shaded in for low, and a figure diagonally striped for high.

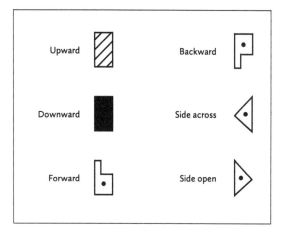

Figure 1.4 Laban space symbols for the six directions (right side)

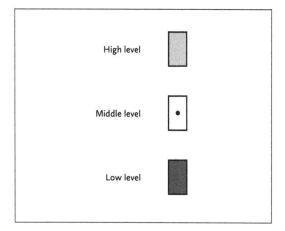

Figure 1.5 Laban's denotation of levels

If we add together the directional symbols with their shading, we have Figure 1.6.

Knowing precisely where one is in space is crucial for movement skill. The more precision,

the higher level of skill possible, because orientation in space is related to gravity and gravity as we know is a force to be reckoned with!

In therapeutic work we may be working with restoring and improving balance in someone elderly or injured. We may be working with someone trying to improve physical performance of an action, from simply picking up and carrying groceries after a lower-extremity injury, to learning to land a flip, to riding, running, or sledding faster. Refining awareness of where the entire body is in space, and where its parts are as we coordinate them throughout the intricacies of movement phrase will improve our motor efficiency.

These baseline somatic practices can be used across the board and can be points of departure for more pointed exploration centered on a specific task, skill acquisition, or improvement of body use.

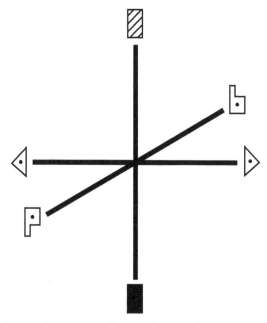

Figure 1.6 Dimensional cross of axes with notations

SOMATIC PRACTICES FOR UNDERSTANDING THE BODY'S "GEOGRAPHY"   31

SOMATIC PRACTICE: Exploring the felt sense of orientation in space through the dimensional cross of axes

1. Begin standing in the anatomical position or in Mountain Pose. Feel the verticality of your uprightness. Imagine the vertical axis arising from the earth between your feet and meeting your torso at the pelvic floor. Locate it traveling through your torso, neck, and out the tip of the top of your head. Did you do any adjustments to your posture or position as you sensed the location of this axis?

2. The vertical axis gives us the experience of the two directions of up and down. Can you feel each one? One is fully away from the earth and the other is fully toward it.

3. Now, using your whole body or choosing a body part like your hand, allow yourself to investigate rising upward away from gravity. What do you need to do to achieve this?

4. Next allow yourself to experience moving toward the earth going downward. What do you need to do for this to happen?

5. Ride the vertical axis and explore moving your body and its parts along this spatial pathway of up to down and up. Certainly you cannot solve this by keeping all the body parts traveling at all times in this singular dimension, so allow for this.

6. What is your experience of the vertical dimension? What does it give to you? When do you find yourself using it in your postural and movement life? Is there anyone you know that seems to "live" or reside in this dimension? Does anyone you know exclude the use of this dimension physically, metaphysically, or metaphorically?

7. Return to the starting position of standing and sense the horizontal dimension. Feel the sides of your body, feel its width. Notice where your body is wider, and where it is narrower. What is your relationship to your experience of width?

8. Now using your entire body, or a part, move side to side. Explore the space as far away from your center as you can to the sides of you without moving from your place. Return to the midline. Feel free to explore.

9. Notice the sense of sidedness, or horizontal dimension. What actions do you do here? When is this dimension important to you in your posture and movement life? What comes up for you here?

10. Return once again to simple standing. Now notice the sagittal dimension. Even though the depth of our body from front to back takes up less space than it did in the other two dimensions just explored, feel this dimension of your volume. When ready, move your entire body, or some part or parts, in this dimension. Explore what comes up for you. When is this dimension used? What is familiar, comfortable, or uncomfortable about it? Notice what you notice.

When observing a client or student, what do you first notice about their inhabitation of space? What does their body posture and position reveal? How would you feel in that space? What is the somatic sense of it? How does the space you occupy affect your awareness of your environment around you? What is cut off from your awareness? What becomes the focus? Explore your response to the space you are in. This is not an interpretation but a somatization, a felt sense of space.

For our purposes, I'm going to introduce some spatial forms and a related scale from Laban's Space Harmony to give you a point of departure for further investigation. We'll return to the dimensional cross of axes and identify its geometric form, then experience one of its movement scales, which Laban called the Defense Scale.

THE OCTAHEDRON

The octahedron is the spatial form that results when connecting the extreme reaches of the six directions of forward, backward, side, side, upward, and downward of the three dimensions.

If one moves primarily along the pathways available in one dimension within this form, one moves from center to periphery and back in one dimension. The joints of the limbs will fold and unfold. If the spine becomes involved, it will make variable movements with the aim of keeping to the singular dimension. The space will inform the mover as well and give a particular felt sense of singular intent within its frame of reference. It should be noted that naturally a three-dimensional form such as the body must inhabit more than one dimension! So some leeway must be given due to the shapes and lengths of one's body and the structures of joints limiting movement possibility. Still, the general spatial motif can be seen and experienced—and that's what we're going for. There is also a particular experience that occurs in relation to primarily one-dimensional movement. It will give a particular felt sense; there is a poetics to it.

SOMATIC PRACTICE: Exploration of moving centrally in the octahedron

Confine yourself to moving your whole body, or its chosen part, to one pathway in space along one singular dimension. This is called central movement, which is movement that generally originates, returns to, or passes through the body's center.

1. Begin with the vertical dimension. Ride the dimension upward and downward in movement. Explore doing it with different parts leading. Feel free to vary the movement in other ways like in timing or intensity. Try this while supporting your body's weight on different supports: on two feet, on one foot, sitting, etc.
2. Next, work with the horizontal dimension, moving side to side in the same way as above. Go as far as you can reach to one side then the other. Try one hand leading,

then the opposite. Do you now see why each side (of left and right) can be called side open and side across?
3. Now explore the sagittal dimension, moving forward and backward. Use your whole body or just one limb, explore as you like. Move centrally, passing through your body's center, along this third dimension.
4. Now allow yourself to move in and out along any of these three pathways from center to the end of your reach space and back to center. This is called central movement.

What is your experience of yourself as you move in this way? How does this affect your thinking, your breathing? When is this space used by you in your posture, gesture and movement life? How does it feel? What does it mean to you?

Octahedral movement

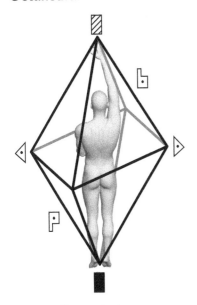

Figure 1.7 The octahedron

Movement in the octahedron can also be done on its periphery. This is done by reaching to the limit of the kinesphere along any of the three dimensions, say to the forward middle direction of the sagittal dimension, and then moving from there to the limit of the kinesphere in a different dimension, say to the left side of the horizontal dimension, and so forth. This is peripheral movement, and it will have its own distinct felt sense as opposed to central movement (Figure 1.7).

SOMATIC PRACTICE: Moving peripherally in the octahedron

With one hand, explore tracing the borders of the octahedron. Move from point to point along the peripheral pathway of an imaginary octahedron framing your body. Using your right hand, explore moving from forward middle to place high, to back middle, to place low, to side across to forward middle and again to side open. Keep your hand moving from one point to the next, never coming into center or passing into the space within the geometric form. What is your experience?

MOVEMENT SCALES

A movement scale is a series of directional changes made by the whole body, a body part, or body parts. It gives us a very good way to explore and experience the differences in one-, two-, and three-dimensional use of space. This in turn gives an understanding of how the dimensionality of the movement done affects the body's tissues, such as the joints, the connective tissue, and the organs. From this experiential understanding we can create therapeutic movements designed to specifically impact target tissues in specific ways.

(When several body parts move along a scale it is considered a chord!) Placing this work of creating movements with target tissues for therapeutic purpose in a yogic context, we are creating therapeutic *vinyasa*.

Vinyasa in its contemporary use refers to yoga postures strung together by movement or yoga-based body positions that include movement. In Sanskrit *vi* refers to creating something for a specific purpose. *Nyasa* refers to doing something that is organized in a meaningful progression.

So, using the idea of creating a specific set of actions to do with a specific purpose would be to create therapeutic *vinyasa* in yoga therapy. Knowing what effect a movement will likely have on target tissues can be grounded in experiential exploration.

A common myth about the invention of yoga postures was that masters discovered them while in states of sublime awareness that included heightened sensitivity to the flow of energy and the cellular intelligence of the body. As practitioners we can spread our fledgling wings and explore our own microcosmic body to feel the effects of movements on our tissues with our own inner sensing apparatus. Guided by their insights, through scripture and oral teachings, we also can respectfully modify for a unique therapeutic purpose, and design based on our own direct experience. This is done with awareness and utmost care, with respectful consideration of what we have been taught.

SOMATIC PRACTICE: Moving in the Defense Scale to experience space

Using the right hand, begin by reaching to forward middle. This is your starting position. To begin the scale:

1. Move your hand peripherally to place high overhead.
2. Then centrally through your center (as best you can) to place low.
3. Then move diagonally side across middle level.
4. Then through center at this level to side open.
5. Then move peripherally back to middle.
6. And return to the starting place moving centrally to forward middle.

You've just done Laban's Defense Scale. Repeat it several times if you like to get the feel of it. To really feel what the movement does to your body, see if you can keep your body's center of mass, your pelvis, generally facing forward the entire time. You'll notice you then will need to do more twisting and shaping in your torso, and it will demand more of your joints.

What did you notice? Can you reverse the scale using your left hand? What would it be like to use your whole body, moving as fully as you can in each direction in space? Can you also do this just with your awareness, locating space outside of your body while sitting or standing in one place? Why do you suppose Laban called this the Defense Scale?

Two other spatial forms are commonly used to explore the richness of attention to space in movement: the icosahedron, which is a joining together of the spatial tensions in the three cardinal planes, and the cube, which is very useful for designing movements for the proximal joints: the shoulders and hips.

THE PLANES AND THE ICOSAHEDRON

When we combine two dimensions we arrive at a plane. A plane has four directional spatial stresses. In anatomical terms, planes are seen as bisecting the body. To study the body and visualize the structures within it, anatomists use the idea of planes to assist observational orientation. The planes have several names. We will favor the movement-oriented terms: vertical plane, sagittal plane, and horizontal plane. The median, or mid-sagittal plane, is a type of sagittal plane that bisects the body's right and left sides.

Moving in each of the planes gives an experience of the body's occupation and use of two-dimensional space. Even though we exist in three-dimensional space, the spatial pulls or tensions of two-dimensional space give a unique experience. Laban combined the far reaches of the three planes to form the 20-sided icosahedron as a spatial form from within which movement could be explored (Figure 1.8).

Because of the geometry of the icosahedron, scales arising there can take the mover to mid-range space so that the mover slices the space between center and periphery. This is where a great deal of movement in daily life takes place.

So icosahedral movement is a good choice, for instance in designing movement for return to activities of daily living after surgery or in joints of limbs.

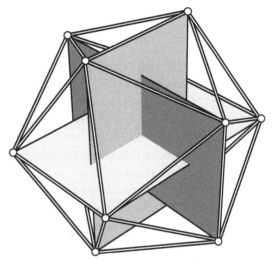

Figure 1.8 The planes and the icosahedron

THE CUBE

In addition, Laban used the cube as a geometric form within which to explore the idea of three equal spatial tensions. Movers are centered within the spatial form and reach to the corners of the cube. In doing so, they experience the equal pull of three dimensions. For instance, with the right hand, reach to the upper right corner of an imaginary cube of which you picture yourself standing in the center. The three spatial stresses are side, as you move sideways from center, forward, and upward. Three equal pulls.

SOMATIC PRACTICE: Moving in the cube

1. Imagine you are standing within a cube. Now try moving around the corners of the top of your cube. Move your hand to right forward high, left forward high, left back high, and right back high.
2. Now try the lower corners: right forward low, left forward low, right back low, and left back low. These move your hand around the corners of the cube at a low level.
3. Remember, you continue to face forward, keeping the front of the pelvis mainly forward as you move. This is called your facing. The cube gives us diagonal movement that has three equal spatial tensions or pulls into diagonal corners. Move from

one diagonal, say right forward high, to its opposite, left back low. Notice that the movement now slices through the cube on a perfect diagonal. Move along the diagonal paths (you have to adjust your body as you are in the center!). Can you feel that this requires some rotation through the torso and some folding and unfolding of the limb joints? What else do you notice?

Exploring space through Laban's Space Harmony, or simply experiencing one's physical use of space throughout one's day, gives us a sense not only of where we tend to be, but how our inhabitation of the space around us makes us feel. We can claim that this is so. But being able to describe and even notate it provides evidence.

For example, my client John's head is always held forward and down. His back and neck are painfully tight, he has tinnitus and jaw pain, and his voice gets hoarse by day's end. He's often overfocused on what's before him. If you ask him to stand up straight his head remains forward and low. His tissues support this posture, and this posture, unfortunately, supports his inability to take a deep full breath.

Working spatially with John may not be your first thought initially as a yoga therapist. It may be to give him some gentle chest openers and some complete breath practices. And that sounds like a good plan, but *where* do those practices take him in space? They take him into more space. What do they provide? They provide a fuller capacity to use the space in and around his body.

CLINICAL APPLICATION FOR THE PHYSICAL SHEATH AND BEYOND

In working to solve presenting issues for clients on the various *koshic* levels, orientation is crucial ground for any progress. Knowing where one is in space in the field of gravity is the somatic basis of our ability to orient. The way we organize to cope with the basic features of our environment becomes an important platform for all other learning. The somatic study of space, although at first seemingly esoteric and not clinically oriented, is ultimately practical and applicable to a great range of disability and its subsequent rehabilitation. Space is not so very abstract. We think in its terms all the time. We use phrases like "forward thinking." We say we are "bending over backward," and ask, "Whose side are you on?" We share that we are feeling "up" or "down." Deals go sideways, we go off on tangents, and we sometimes get spaced out. Space is also very much part of our first experience.

In clinical application we can observe body parts moving in space. How and where is the weight being transferred in a movement, like in taking a step forward? How is the person's center of gravity being propelled over their bases of support? Are they organized well enough around their axis? If not, what is preventing that and what is the path to change for them? Stopping this down in our experience, we are looking at *where* body parts are moving in relation to one another. We're perceiving them in terms of their spatial relationships and whether where they move in space is functional or needs guidance for improvement.

The premise of this book, and of somatic practice in general, is that an experiential base gives a richer, more nuanced and deeper understanding of the application of yoga practice. Deepening into one of the main contexts of our existence, that of an experience of space, is going to be a huge underpinning for all that follows.

In approaching orthopedic issues of the physical sheath we look to how the body areas in question move. Do they move with ease?

Thinking in terms of space, what space does the body part take up? What are its dimensions and in what planes does it exist? When moving, does the movement go where it ought to go? Is there enough differentiation or mobility where there naturally should be? Or is there too much? Also where is the support for the movement in the field of gravity? Does this seem efficient? Is the body organized around its axis? If a part is in question, is the movement organized well spatially so weight travels well through tissues designed for it or is this not the case? Where in space is this off kilter? Where does the weight go in the space the body inhabits—too far forward on the foot? And then why is that? Is this because there is not enough movement at the ankle joint, or because there is not enough support through the toe knuckle, or both? And which came first?

When looking at how the movement is organized, we look for efficiency. Does the initiation and sequencing of the movement seem roundabout, extraneous, strenuous, or precarious? In answering these, and other questions, what we are observing in our assessment is the body and its parts moving *in space.*

I think in terms of space when I seek to design a remedy as well. Perhaps I decide that the inhibition of full dorsiflexion at the ankle must be due to a buildup of scar tissue around the Achilles tendon. I still need to think spatially to direct the heel downward and the talus back and down as I direct the distal end of the tibia forward. The more precise I can be with the tissues and their movements in space, the more pointed my remedial therapeutic *vinyasa* for the ankle will be! I use a deep awareness of space to repattern the movement organization as well as the tissue engagement for support in rehabilitating the ankle.

Certainly, space can be expressive. When we see someone slumped forward, their chest depressed downward, head drooping, a felt sense of mood or emotion through our own mirror neurons and sense of empathy is engendered. A basis of sensing and understanding the fundamental experiences of space gives us greater range in relating to others in their bodily inhabitation and use of space at the mental and emotional sheaths. But this is a topic for another chapter.

EXPERIENCING THE TERMS OF POSITION AND DIRECTION

From the fundamental experience of knowing where in space my body parts are and how they each relate in the field of gravity I can begin to repattern faulty bodily use and develop and refine movement skill.

The anatomical terms of position and direction describe relationships between aspects of the body. These are oriented in space using the anatomical position: body standing erectly, limbs extended, with the palms of the hands forward. Beginning with the anatomical position, these terms provide a vocabulary with which we can talk about the relationship of the body parts in terms of the space they occupy. Exploring these terms bodily with sensation and movement deepens our understanding of these terms, making them more memorable.

Beyond this, it develops our ability to feel the location of the anatomical features within our own body. I'm able to locate within my body aspects of my anatomy in relation to other aspects. This integrates the anatomical knowledge of terms and descriptions with spatial awareness within my body, along with whatever my inner sensing capability is, and with my ability to visualize. Also, I think proportionally and sense the size of my own body's anatomical features. This becomes the basis for translating all of learning through these various modes of understanding to the bodies of others. I'll be better able to do so once I have felt and visualized and mapped the anatomical features of my own body. It is proportional and "proxemical" thinking; proportional in that I am sensing the size and position, and proxemical, from proxemics, the study of spatial relationships, in that I am becoming aware of how the various attributes of my body exist and function in relation to one another in space.

I liken developing this type of awareness to knowing where your neighbors live in your apartment building. If I am home in my second-floor rear apartment and think of my neighbor who lives on the fourth floor in the front, let's call it 4A, I can sense outside of myself, based on having been to the apartment, where in space that person will be. I have a good idea of it spatially. If I were able to throw a magic ball hard enough through the walls and up two flights, I'd be able to aim it to reach my neighbor's apartment because I have a sense of where it exists in external space. This is the translation I mean when I say once we can locate items and features of our own anatomy, our own apartment as it were, we can begin to translate that process to sensing and then imaging beyond our body boundaries into space.

SOMATIC PRACTICE: Terms of position and direction somatization

We'll explore the terms of position and direction through a process of visualization and inner sensing and, if you are inclined, movement (Figure 1.9). As in all this work, please allow your curiosity to guide your exploration as well as my direction.

- cranial, superior, rostral—being closer to the head (the cranium) or higher
- anterior, ventral—being located more in front of something else
- posterior, dorsal—being located behind or more in back of something else
- medial—being closer to the midline than something else
- lateral—being further from the midline, usually to the sides
- proximal—only used for the limbs; being closer to the root of the limb or core of the body than something else
- distal—only used for the limbs; being father away from the limb root or core of the body
- caudal, inferior—tailward or closer to the lower part of the body; used with the torso only
- superficial—on the body's surface

- deep—further from the surface
- ipsilateral—means "on the same side"
- contralateral—means "on the opposite side."

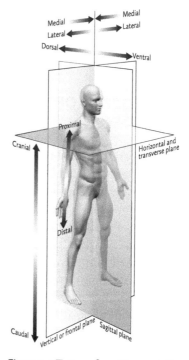

Figure 1.9 Terms of position and direction

1. Please lie comfortably on the floor in as close to the anatomical position as is comfortable. Begin by becoming aware of "place center" which, for this exercise, is located a tad below the navel in the center of your body in terms of depth front to back. Take a moment to sense this location in your body. Assign to this area the role of anchor or homebase as a point of reference for your exploration.

2. Now focus on, and focus includes feeling in your body, the space your body takes up headward of your center. This is called cranial, which of course refers to your cranium, i.e., the skull around your brain. It is also called superior, which generally means above. Whatever is above your center is superior to it. Sometimes the term "rostral" is also used. Rostral is from the Latin *rostrum* and refers to a beak. Our bipedal stance causes our anatomy to make a 90-degree turn, moving our nose and mouth forward instead of directly upward. In humans the term indicates the front of the brain. So, when discussing the head, rostral will mean forward or anterior, to the front; but here, with the entire body, it can be interchanged with superior. These terms are used to show relationships.

3. Now notice the location of your heart in your chest. Do your best to sense its location. Notice its location above your pelvis. Your heart is superior to your pelvis. It is rostral to it. It is cranial to it, although that sounds weird.

4. Choose another organ above your pelvis. Notice your sense of it being above or superior. Now, if you like, initiate movement above your center and allow yourself to move in any way you want. It is fine if you end up moving more than the area just above your pelvic center.

5. Return to awareness of your pelvic center.

Now become aware of the space the body takes up lower than this area. This is inferior, or caudal. Caudal is from the Latin for tail, *cauda*.

6. And just for the sake of exploring the terms in a way that makes them very useful, please locate and sense into the space that is occupied by your brain. Now sense the very top of your head, or the most superior place in your body. Sense your heart. Notice that it is inferior to your brain, while it is also superior to your pelvic center. These terms help us locate body parts and areas in relation to one another in space.

7. Here are some other terms for exploration:
   • anterior or ventral—being located more in front of something else
   • posterior or dorsal—being located behind, or more in back of something else.

We'll start standing for this next part. See if you can sense the division of the real estate of your body in terms of what is front and what is back. The dividing line would be somewhere around the middle of your ears, sides of your ribs and hips and knees, right down to the large knobs (greater malleoli) of your ankle bones.

8. Now sense the front of the body, the anterior portion. This is also called ventral, which is based on the Latin for stomach. What is the area like? What do you notice?

9. Now sense the back of the body, the posterior or dorsal portion. What is this like? The same relational use of these terms applies. You can say your stomach is ventral or anterior to your kidneys, and conversely your kidneys are posterior or dorsal to your stomach, although posterior is more commonly used here.

10. Now allow yourself to initiate movement from the anterior parts of your body. What

does it feel like to embody your body in this way? Is it familiar? Does it have a feeling to it? Let go of this and switch your awareness to the posterior aspect. Move from there. What does that bring forth in your awareness? Allow yourself to play as long as you like with these various locations and relationships.

11. Next feel your body's midline, separating left from right side. They almost match fully except for some organs. A specialized plane called the median plane is the border between one side of your body and the other. It bisects your body's sides. There is so much important to the sensing of this central line; take your time here.

12. Medial refers to anything that is closest to this plane in your body. Its counter is lateral, which refers to anything further to the sides. Your ribs are lateral to your spine. Conversely your spine is medial to your ribs.

13. Here's another one: feel that your kidneys are lateral to your midline, but your skin on the sides of your torso is lateral to your kidneys. Now locate this going inward. Most lateral is the skin. Then locate the more medial kidneys and, medial to that, your midline and spine. Feel the difference. Move initiating first from parts of your body that are medial, then try lateral initiations. What do you notice?

Proximal and distal relate to these as well but refer to your limbs. Proximal refers to being closer to the root of the limb and distal, like something in the distance, is further away.

There are two more terms that are very useful in hands-on and imaging practices in which you sense into the body, either your own or another person's. They are "superficial" and "deep."

14. Begin by feeling the skin and the surfaces of your body. Then move your attention inward a slight bit, no more than an inch. Feel this area of your body. What kind of information do you find yourself noticing? Then as you like, move further in, with your awareness. If this is at first too much to track, begin with your arms. Gradually bring your awareness inward to the deeper tissues of bones and where the marrow would be. What do you notice? Are you able to concentrate and keep your awareness there? If you like, try this with your legs. Then your torso, then your neck and finally the head. Is there any area that is less accessible to your awareness? What comes to the screen of your mind?

15. If you like, orient your body to the different planes in space. Stand in the vertical plane. Then bend forward from the hips and reach out to the sides. Perhaps, if you can, lift a leg behind to occupy the horizontal plane. Then, find the parts of you that can move readily into the space behind and in front of you while facing forward—this is moving into the sagittal plane.

You may at first think that this is child's play and not for adults, who can easily learn terminology and remember names. While this may be true about memorization, embodying the concepts, feeling them in your body, gives a clear experience of the terms and not only helps you remember them, but, more importantly, gives you a somatic sense that can be translated to observation of others, hands-on palpation and body work skills, and a basis for designing therapeutic *vinyasa* for clearer articulation in movement, resulting in better functioning of bodies other than your own.

PALPATION AND VISUALIZATION

Palpation is used in a variety of approaches to working with and caring for the body. From western medical diagnosis to sensing the flow of cerebrospinal fluid to feeling for energetic abundance and dearth, reading the body through touch is a direct means of perceiving what is happening in its tissues and beyond. Developing palpatory skill is acquired by practice. In our work we use palpation diagnostically as well as in re-education through tissue communication. This involves not only palpatory sensitivity, but also knowledge of the territory under our hands. To use palpation to learn anatomy is an excellent way to begin to learn to read the body.

From this beginning of making sense of what is under our hands, we learn to feel for anatomical structures. Once this is in play, we can then go on to fitting the information we get into the diagnostic framework of the therapeutic model within which we are practicing.

Even so, we must in any approach remain open to the impressions we receive through our touch. We do this while at the same time we layer our idea of what and where the anatomical features are so we can create a felt sense of what is observed through our touch.

Taking this one step further, we may also sense in our own body to locate what is within the body of another. This self-referencing and comparison can give greater ability to locate deeper tissues in touch and over time can lead to more subtle recognition of the states of the tissues themselves within our own body and in the tissues of others.

Palpating the bony landmarks in standing alignment

Alignment is a uniquely personal story of how each of us uses our skeletal scaffolding in stillness and in movement to contend with the constant force of gravity. Each story features the use of our human structure over time as we manage the challenges we face throughout life. In alignment we want our well-orchestrated skeleton to be the main weight-bearing structure. Guiding this body use is a feature of hands-on adjustments in yoga practice, especially in the basis of all standing poses, *Tadasana* (Mountain Pose) or Simple Standing Pose.

In any structure, mechanical balance occurs when the forces acting on the structure are in balance. This produces a state of equilibrium. A pyramid, for example, is a very stable mechanically balanced structure. It exemplifies the features that make for stability, such as: a broad base of support, a central axis of gravity, with the center of weight close to its base, and an even distribution of weight around its axis. Of course, a pyramid is not very movable. Our body features a very moveable spine and a unique arrangement of limbs balancing in locomotion on merely two of them. This presents an intriguing structural problem for our bodies to solve when ease of stance in alignment is sought.

A VIEW OF THE BODY'S WEIGHT-BEARING STRUCTURE

The body's structure employs both compressional stress (a squeezing pressure) and tensile stress (a pulling pressure) to bear weight. There are three *main* designs in the human skeletal system in which weight:

1. *sits* (compressional)
2. is *braced* (compressional) or
3. *hangs* (tensile).

The structure of our spine and human form is not built solely for stability. The spine is a mobile structure that carries a lot of weight which we ask, at times, to act in a stable manner. In yoga practice we move and position the spine in stability in a wide variety of planes and positions. When working with standing alignment it is useful to consider the body in terms of three major body weights and five spinal curves. Representing the central axis of our structure we can envision a plumb line running from the center of the top of the head through the center of our stance between our feet (Figure 1.10).

Tapping yourself on the center of the top of the head can stimulate awareness of your plumb line.

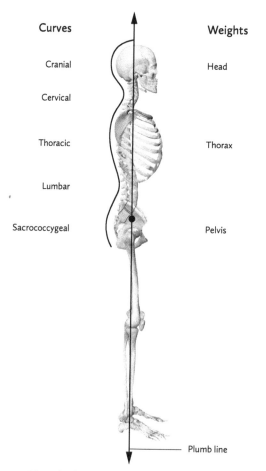

Figure 1.10 Three body weights, five spinal curves, and plumb line

SOMATIC PRACTICE: Palpating the bony landmarks in standing alignment

This one requires a partner. Ask permission of your partner and let them know they can tell you to stop at any time and to please share anything they would like to share as you work. Have your partner stand in Mountain Pose or a simple standing position and observe them from the side.

1. First, look for the alignment of these body parts to fall along the plumb line.

The bony landmarks:

- the center of the ear
- the greater tubercle of the humerus bone at the shoulder
- the center of the side of the ribcage at around sixth or seventh rib
- the greater trochanter of the hip
- the center of the crease of the knee
- the greater malleolus of the ankle.

2. With awareness of the firmness of your own bones in your fingers, begin by palpating:

    a. The top of the head. See if you can find the very top of the skull of your partner and apply gentle pressure to stimulate awareness of the plumb line in standing alignment.

    b. At the ear allow your fingertips to touch the skull around the outside of the ear to assess the alignment of the head. Ear size can vary greatly, so locate the center of the ear where it goes into the skull and use this as your landmark.

    c. Continue to use touch to press into the tissues as you travel down the side of the body to locate the skeletal features and assess whether or not these landmarks align along the vertical dimension of your partner's plumb line.

GOING THROUGH THE TISSUES

Learning to see into the body through touch is a skill that develops with practice. As the saying goes, palpation is learned by doing palpation. We know that the map is not the territory, but a good map sure goes a long way toward familiarity with it. To feel into the body as it were, that is, to perceive more deeply than the skin and superficial surfaces, we must project our awareness deeper into the body. Doing so we have to open to the impressions that come and at the same time, search for what the map instructs us as to what will be there. I've heard of exercises in which masters of palpation invite their students to place a nickel or dime under a magazine and then invite their students to locate and describe which coin they feel through touch (Chaitow, 1991). To the novice this may seem an impossible task; to the experienced practitioner, a worthwhile challenge. One time one of my teachers, Bonnie Bainbridge Cohen, was working with a baby. As she held the baby in her lap, cradling its body between her forearms, with hands gently holding and moving the baby's skull, she was asked what she was feeling in her hands. Her remark surprised the inquirer when she responded that in one finger she was "in" the nervous system, in another finger in the blood, another in the cerebrospinal fluid, and so forth.

Early on in my work of using my hands as diagnostic tools, I had the experience of sitting with other body workers of various backgrounds who found sport in sensing the legs of a wooden table at which we were gathered. With hands on the table, eyes closed, I found myself feeling "the give" of the parts not directly supported by a leg and tracking the increasing density of pressure when my awareness through my hands approached a table leg's vertical thrusting against gravity. All this through the grain of the table surface where I was seated.

The somatic practice that follows is my version of how I perceive within the body through the sense of touch. It is based on two types of hands-on training I've had the honor of studying: Shaitsu-Amma as taught by Dr. DoAnn Kaneko, and Body-Mind Centering® created by Bonnie Bainbridge Cohen. I've been doing and teaching this technique in this fashion for several decades, so it may more resemble the strokes of my use than any original bearing.

SOMATIC PRACTICE: Going through the tissues hands-on

You'll need a partner for this practice. You and your partner can decide to explore any part of the body; if you are not sure, try the forearm as it is a relatively simple part of the body anatomically speaking. Then find a "map" or two (or more) in the form of an image, diagram, anatomical drawing, model, or the like of the area you've chosen. Look at the images and consider the anatomical features like a landscape you'll be visiting. Get your bearings; get a sense of the neighborhood if you will.

1. When you begin, start with the sense being present. Make contact and just "be" for a moment.
2. Next, allow yourself to be open to what you notice under your hand or hands. Just as you might sense location in space, allow your awareness to go more deeply into the tissues. What do you notice?
3. If you saw a specific thing, such as a bone like the radius, or perhaps, if you chose the torso, an organ, allow your attention to scan for where you might expect it to be. Notice what you notice. Remain focused and allow yourself to be open to your awareness through your hands.

Sometimes it can be helpful to locate within your own body the tissue or exact structure, i.e., your own radius, or kidney, or whatever it is, while you are searching for the tissue in someone else. A sort of resonance at times can be found. Also, at times, dialoguing with your partner can be useful as some will feel your intention and meet you with their awareness in the target tissue you are looking for.

4. Once a target tissue or anatomical structure is contacted, explore its qualities, size, dimensions, and other features of interest that may appear to your perception.

We'll leave off in this exercise with location and contact, but next could be an assessment of the felt sense of what you have contacted. And if you and your partner were to decide on an additional purpose for the touch, after assessment, you would then begin that agenda.

5. When you return to the surface, come back out with attention on the tissues you are perceiving as you return to the surface. Spend a moment just being present on the surface before ending contact.

With practice you may find this type of palpation exploration enhances your ability to assess what is happening with different tissues such as muscles, tendon, bones, fascia, and organs. We leave off prior to assessment and educational, remedial touch here, but as you explore you may begin to see, implicit in this approach, an ability to support deeper tissues of the body through touch with what they appear to need.

TRACING THE BONES TO EXPERIENTIALLY UNDERSTAND SUPPORT AND SPATIAL CLARITY

Typically, when learning anatomy, we see images on a page with some description. To truly be able to embody this, it can be very useful to use the sense of touch when possible. Beyond simply learning the locations, being implicitly aware of how the spatial integrity and scaffold-like form of our skeleton provides leverage in movement can be instructive in designing repatterning experiences for students and clients.

I first learned to trace the bones while studying Shiatsu-Amma. It was done for the purpose of locating acupoints, which required a sense of understanding the client's proportions. The locations of acupoints were found by locating a bony landmark and then measuring by the number of finger-widths of the individual receiving the treatment. Body-Mind Centering® also explores the skeletal system through touch, imagery, movement, and inner sensing and feeling, the latter two of which Bonnie Bainbridge Cohen differentiates. My experience of sensing is of my mental awareness looking for and finding what

is to be experienced; as Bonnie has said, I am recording it in my nervous system. Feeling for me is the resultant bifurcation of impressions and associations I get from a targeted inquiry based on my attention to a body area or tissue.

Anatomical pictures provide the maps to the territory. Then palpation of a body area is undertaken, with the investigation focused on a sense of open presence to experience. It should be noted that Bonnie has written a book titled *Sensing, Feeling, and Action* (2012). And for me, the title suggests the process. To sense, then to have a felt response, and then to move, which for me provides integration of what was discovered into the ongoing refinement of my embodiment as the matrix of movement.

SOMATIC PRACTICE: Tracing the bones of the hand

In this exploration we'll focus on the bones of the hand because you can easily do this alone. This is also a good place to begin with a partner. Another good starting point for partner work is the scapula. It is somewhat less personal as your partner is facing away and the upper back is an area of social touch, and much of the bone is tactually available, though some of the scapular edges may need to be imagined.

1. Begin by finding a few good images that show the bones of the hand from potentially more than one point of view. If there's specific points of interest, like an area of discomfort or injury, or just a curiosity, like how voluminous joint capsules are, find the best images you can for them.

2. Feel the hand that will be the focus of the work. Move it as you normally do. Experience its form, tone, density, and whatever comes to the screen of your mind—notice what you notice. If you like, you could jot down some descriptors: it feels like a soft watery balloon, it feels denser in

the middle, or whatever. You might also draw your impression like an impressionist painter. This is not an anatomical drawing of your hand, but of your experiential impression of your hand.

3. Now begin with the tip of the thumb, and using your anatomical image "maps," use your thumb and index finger of the other hand to press on the sides of the tip of the thumb till you can feel the firmness of the bone underneath. Continue to explore with pressing and squeezing motions. Look with your awareness for the shape of the bone as it is pictured. And, since you are doing this with yourself, pay attention to what you feel as well in the explored hand. Notice what comes to you. See if you can get a three-dimensional image of the bone and bony area.

4. Continue onto the joint, checking in with the anatomy "maps" of the terrain you're exploring. Then follow this process going from bone to joint up into the metacarpals

and then finally into the carpals or wrist bones themselves.

5. Repeat with each finger.

6. Finally, using your anatomy maps, examine your carpal bones. It may be useful to place the images in the same orientation as your hand, and then explore which bones you are able to palpate and possibly move or wiggle gently. Finding the ends of the radius and ulna bones can help you locate the carpal bones close to the wrist joint. You may notice that the wrist joint is not a simple space between one bone and the next but is made up of several bones: the radius and ulna on the forearm side, and the triquetrum, lunate, and scaphoid on the hand side. You may also be able to locate the articular disc between the ulna and the triquetrum bone. The pea-sized moveable pisiform bone, located on the palmar side of the triquetrum, may make itself known as well.

7. Once you have investigated the bones of the hand to your satisfaction, pause. Allow yourself to notice whatever you notice about the explored hand now. How does it present itself on the screen of your mind? What impressions do you now have that weren't there before? Move the hand and notice how the movement feels. How would you describe or picture it? See if you would like to make a sketch, write some descriptors down, create a movement, or in some other way record your experience.

SOMATIC PRACTICE: Sculptural modeling to further conceptualize and explore the three-dimensional relationships of body forms

Sculpting anatomical structures can be an excellent way to understand them more fully. You might wonder how this is a somatic practice. It becomes one when you bring your awareness into your own body as a guiding relationship for the subject you'll be making. You may ask a friend to help you locate something that can be palpated in part at least, like a spinous process. Or you may use anatomical images as your source.

We're going to make the 12th thoracic vertebra (Figure 1.11).

To begin, find as many images of the structure you've chosen to model as you can. See if you can find them pictured from a variety of angles. Also find ones that show its location in the body. Then sit or lie down and see if you can locate the structure in your own body. Can you initiate movement from it or from the region of the body in which it exists? Change positions and track where it goes and how your movements affect it. What forces flow through it as you move? What else do you notice? When you have spent some time exploring the structure in your own body to your satisfaction, gather your materials and go to work!

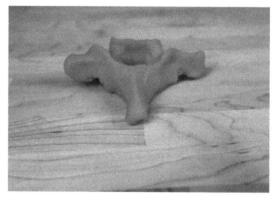

Figure 1.11 The 12th thoracic vertebra

You can use modeling clay, Play-Doh, or make your own. If you want to DIY it, simply mix together:

- ¾ cup water (180g/6.5oz)
- ¾ cup salt (215g/7.5oz)
- 2 cups flour (240g/8.5oz).

Knead this mixture until it forms a ball (add a tad more water if needed) and you're ready! This is self-hardening, so once you've made the model and it dries, it will keep its form.

This exploration of modeling is particularly useful in understanding the difference between the cervical, thoracic, and lumbar vertebrae and helps to get a fuller sense of how they hold the weight share, as well as the delicacy of the entire spinal structure. Any bones are good candidates for modeling. Shaping the bones around the sinuses of the head, or making a sternum with the manubrium, body, and xiphoid process gives a wealth of information as to the size of this important series of bones covering the heart and lungs. If you choose to make this series of bones as well, once your model has hardened, search for a found object, such as a piece of fruit or stone the approximate size of the heart. The experience of creating these forms is not only memorable but can also be very edifying.

SKETCHING TO LEARN NAME, LOCATION, AND RELATIONSHIP

Attempting to draw the features of an anatomical part or area can at first seem daunting. Here it's important to remember that this is not for the sake of the product but for the experiential process of doing so and what can be learned. As in modeling, an easy point of entry is the skeletal system, but any part of interest will yield good results in terms of better understanding. The learning is in the process of doing.

As above, using several images to get a sense of the subject, say a left collarbone, is a good start. If the body area is palpable, doing self-palpation is next. If not, using the practice "Going through the tissues," or simply sensing and visualizing within the body to locate the subject, should be done in a quiet moment without interruption.

Another possible subject choice is to draw a more complex body area like the hand, or the entire rib cage. Drawing the digestive system with the placement of the surrounding and supporting organs like the spleen and pancreas can also be worthwhile. These types of drawings help us more fully understand the proportion and relationship of the various aspects involved and open new areas of curiosity as we work to place the parts on the page. It is almost impossible not to include something of one's own experiential anatomy when working this way. Graph paper can be used if preferred to help with proportion.

SOMATIC PRACTICE: Drawing a body part or area

1. Begin with a set-up of blank paper or graph paper as you choose. Many students find that anatomical sketching becomes a relaxing and rewarding pastime, so having a sketch book for this may be a choice as well.
2. Choose the body part or area to be drawn.

Locate more than one map of the item or territory you will draw. Spend time letting your curiosity guide you. Focus on what you are curious about. How big is one aspect in relation to another? What is the connection like between things? See what draws your attention.

3. If possible, palpate the area while sensing into it to get a feel for dimensions and other qualities. As you do this, see if you can visualize the part or area in question.

4. Now simply allow yourself to draw what you recall from your explorations. If you're a bit squeamish about drawing, I recommend setting a time like ten minutes, and committing to working on your drawing for that time. See what you can do. You can check back and forth with your images at hand, erase, start over; it matters not.

5. Once you've finished, if you like, see if you can label any of the details of your image. Or just leave it as is. Then once again sense into your body for the subject you've just drawn. Notice what is now apparent to you. What is clearer? Where are your new questions? What might you like to draw next?

This exercise focuses on drawing the anatomical features of a subject such as the collarbone, or an area like the rib cage in general (see Figure 1.12). A further way you can focus this exercise is to add your own felt sense to the image. Rather than trying to get it right, as in making a recognizable anatomical drawing, zero in again on the part you've chosen but bring to the foreground your experience of the anomalies of your own embodiment of that part. What are the features of your own body that are perhaps different from the images you have collected? Is the bone shorter? Longer? Thicker? Feel into your body and begin again drawing the subject you've chosen, but this time focus more on your own physical experience than on "getting it right" or matching the images or descriptions. This may end up looking more like a cartoon or modern art image than a realistic representation. Then reflect on what the end drawing looks like to you. What does it say about your relationship to this tissue? What do you notice?

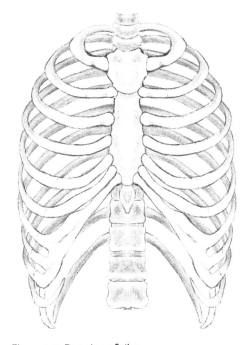

Figure 1.12 Drawing of ribs

DRAWING ON THE BODY CANVAS

This method includes two ways of embodying the anatomy of focus. First is to translate the anatomical learning, say of the origin and insertion of a muscle or the like, to a canvas, albeit the canvas is on the human form. The second is "wearing" the drawing in activity. Putting the body in postures and positions as well as moving with the anatomical drawing covering the body will illustrate the location and participation of the subject. Doing this can create a deep awareness of just exactly where that anatomical feature is and what it is all about.

If you wish to make a wearable item that is more lasting and you have a good budget, you can use white or tan canvas and acrylic paint. You can also purchase relatively tight-fitting single-colored clothing to paint. Depending on the body part or area you've chosen, you may need a fair amount of paint and canvas. For a less expensive and more temporary route, simply use white (clear works well too for a different look) unscented trash bags and colored markers.

You'll need a partner for this, and some images as resources as above. To set this up simply place the canvas over the area you wish to draw. You can have your partner hold the canvas or, for where they can't reach or for better stability, use painters' tape and tape it to their adjacent clothes. This could be really any area of the body, except for the face, obviously, if you are using plastic. We often draw the layer of the abdominal muscles. Other great areas for this are the muscles in the forearms and forelegs, and of course there is always the back.

With muscle layers, like those in the back, you can have several canvases prepared. Draw a layer, take this one off and draw the next, and so forth. Then display them next to one another. If you have wall space—which many yoga and wellness studios do—use non-marking wall putty and hang up the images. You will then have a gallery of what you've drawn.

Before displaying the canvases on the wall, have your partner move and walk, or do *asana* or daily activities to study their anatomy in motion. The person wearing the "artwork" can get a good sense of their anatomy and its function in this way as well (Figure 1.13).

I have used this for clients when I've felt it was important for them to understand where an injury was, what tissue was involved, and how their movement was affected by it. Client education is of great importance when self-care and correct use during remedial exercise is the way out of pain and dysfunction.

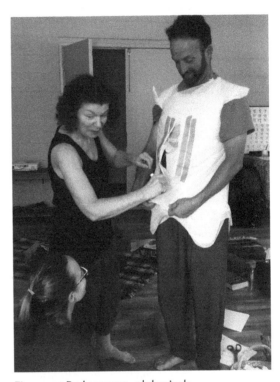

Figure 1.13 Body canvas—abdominals

TAPING THE MUSCLES

Muscle taping is a great way to feel and understand not only the exact location or the span of a muscle, but its line of pull in contraction. As in the practices above, it's good to have on hand a variety of images from different sources. An excellent one for muscle taping is Robert and Judith Stone's *Atlas of Skeletal Muscles* (Stone & Stone, 1999). I prefer drawn images over computer-generated ones, so the older editions are better for this. This is because the computer-generated ones are often less precise when it comes to the muscle attachments.

For this practice you'll need a partner, although you can do some of the leg taping quite well alone (Figure 1.14). You'll also need a variety of colored masking tape. You can buy colored arts and crafts masking tape online or if you have a good hardware store you may be able to find a few different colors of painter's tape, which sticks well and comes off easily. A more expensive version is colored kinesiology tape. This is useful if you wish to keep it on and move around.

Like the body canvas drawing above, have several images on hand to show you exactly where the muscle line goes. Palpate it if superficial, or use "Going through the tissues" to imagine the muscle's pathway inside the body. Then note both ends, the origin and insertion—this will help you aim the line—then tape. If you have a wider muscle, you can choose to fill it in taping according to its structure, i.e., whether it has parallel fibers or pennate ones. Or just get a sense of the line of pull if you want to focus on just one thing.

If you don't have a partner and do have a skeleton, you can tape onto the skeleton. You can do this with a smaller than normal size one too!

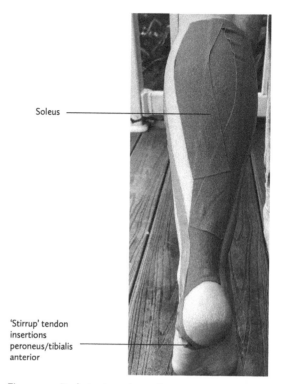

Soleus

'Stirrup' tendon insertions peroneus/tibialis anterior

Figure 1.14 Body taping—lower leg

FOUND OBJECTS THAT ILLUSTRATE ANATOMY AND BIOMECHANICAL FEATURES

Using what you already may have drawn or made as a source for further exploration can be rich and rewarding. When you turn your attention to functionality, to the biomechanics of movement, it can be useful to find ordinary objects that can illustrate a feature of what you are working with. Walk through a hardware store, toy store, or flea market and see what you can find that reminds you of a movement principle in action. Here are some favorites of mine:

- Levers are a no-brainer. Choose from wrenches, shovels, crowbars, and wheelbarrows.
- Mortar and pestles for ball and socket joints; a ball in a cup; an actual ball joint (Figure 1.15).

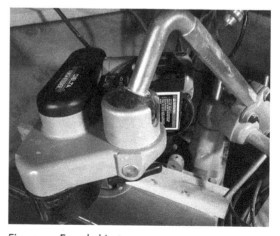

Figure 1.15 Found object

- Pennate muscle: a feather, leaves with veins (Figure 1.16).

- The quadriceps femoris: a tulip!
- A brace or clamp to show the sacral bone between the two ilia.
- Tensegrity toy for babies—to show tensile structures like the arches of the feet and properties of fascia (Figure 1.17).
- Individually wrapped liquorice sticks bundled and wrapped in cling wrap to show muscle fibers covered by fascia (Figure 1.18).
- Squirt chewing gum (gum with gel-like liquid in its center) to show the nucleus pupusa in the spinal disc.
- Mud or cornstarch and water to demonstrate the colloidal property of connective tissue.
- Melt hardened honey to show the thixotropy of tissues (property of heat making them more pliable) (Figure 1.19).

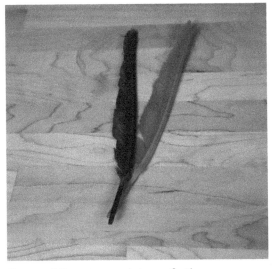

Figure 1.16 Pennate muscle type—feathers

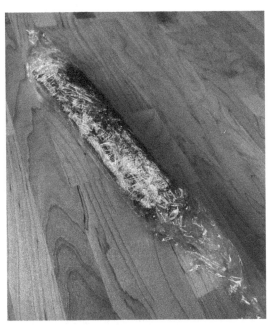

Figure 1.18 Liquorice sticks and cling wrap—muscle fibers and fascia

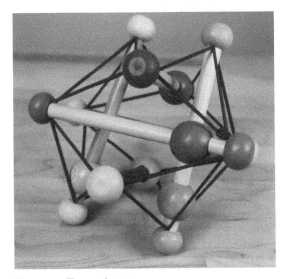

Figure 1.17 Tensegrity toy

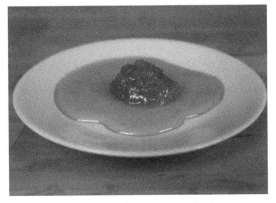

Figure 1.19 Thixotropy of tissues—melting honey

LIVING SCHEMATA: MAKING A MODEL WITH PEOPLE AND PROPS

Another way to access anatomy or anatomical function is to act it out. To do this you most likely won't be able to include all the details of a physiological process or the features of its anatomy, yet you can depict the essence of, say, a chemical exchange or create a reasonable model of a body area on which you'd like to focus. Many science teachers have students act out a reflex arc, or the chemical activity of muscle contraction. This sort of theater of the body is fun and memorable.

Imaging lines of pull in the pelvic floor

For our purposes here, we'll create a simple view of the female pelvic floor. In our training we guide students through a process of drawing the muscles within a diamond-shaped frame representing the borders of the pubic rami, the ischial tuberosities, along the border of the great sacroiliac ligament and the coccyx.

If students are willing, we invite them to sit on a blank piece of paper and map the inferior opening of the pelvic bowl onto the page. One can tilt to the sides and mark the sit bones, then lean back to mark the coccyx. The pubic symphysis can be estimated, dropping one's pencil to the page. Then take the paper out and connect the dots. It is often surprising to see the size of your own pelvic opening opposed to what you thought it would be. Sometimes it will be drawn asymmetrically, or with other anomalies which can be the beginning of interesting further exploration.

SOMATIC PRACTICE: Group modeling of the pelvic floor

Four people are the minimum number to have for this exercise. More are welcome! If you have uncut rolls of resistance bands you can use them. Long pieces of jersey or another stretch fabric work well too.

The first set of participant roles are to define the bony landmarks. One person sits at the place of the coccyx, with two more people a short distance away on each side representing the ischial tuberosities. The fourth person sits opposite the coccyx still further away as the pubic symphysis.

If only using four people, if possible, they can extend their legs to the sides and create a diamond shape to indicate the pelvic bowl and its inferior opening. From this outline the bands or fabric you've chosen can be placed or held (having more than four people can help with this) between them, crossing the space. If you like, you can use an index card and write the names of the muscles you add as a label for them. Begin at the inferior level and work upward into the pelvis.

MOVING TO INTEGRATE LEARNING

In the practice of yoga therapy the end goal of training is for graduates to have skill in the application of their learning and practical experience. Ideally the therapist will not only be able to reproduce protocols they have been exposed to in class but will be able to think on their feet, making their own decisions when met with new and unique situations.

What this requires is integration of learning which is connecting concepts to experience.

This skill in integration is an important aspect of successful therapeutic work. When the body is concerned, movement is the great integrator. Just as the adage in palpation goes—palpation is learned through palpation—the practical skill of integration is learned through integration.

Movement during this sort of somatic investigation helps to integrate learning in two important ways: top-down and bottom-up. Top-down and bottom-up are both strategies for processing and organizing concepts and experience. Moving, sensing, thinking, and feeling dovetail learning in both directions.

Bottom-up, I can begin by simply moving without a focus or objective. Then, as I continue, I may be drawn to a particular feature of my experience, say my footfall, the way my foot contacts the floor as I transfer weight onto it. My curiosity about my experience will lead me to a top-down investigation, say of the bones and how they carry the weight of my body. I may then begin to piece together the relevant elements of the learning on this and related subjects to better map and understand my questions as they emerge. How is my weight being transferred? Does this depend on how long a stride I take? Are my ligaments doing their job? Or whatever it may be, depending on what I am noticing and how the various aspects or anatomy, kinesiology, and movement theory that I've learned are applicable to my quandaries.

A top-down approach of this same content area when explored in movement would begin with my conception of footfall. I would look at and learn about gait and weight transference onto and off the foot. Then I'd get into analyzing what I'm doing, breaking down the different aspects of alignment, push-off, contact with the surface, and the like. I'm moving in a sense to create data for analysis and possible correction.

The layering of information into the felt experience, and felt experience as the ground for investigation, helps students understand the location and the felt sense of the body's functions intimately. Movement amplifies our understanding of how our body is used.

Additionally, movement gives an opportunity to take what has been learned through and in the body locally into the larger matrix of the whole body. And this is how repatterning happens. This is precisely how we *change* through the principles and practice of yoga therapy.

CHAPTER 2

Somatic Practices for Experientially Exploring and Illustrating Physiological Processes

LEARNING BY DOING

By now you know I value learning by doing over pretty much any other way; particularly when what we're trying to achieve in skill in not only meeting another person where they are, but in finding useful ways to facilitate their movement in a healthier, more whole, and wholesome direction.

The collection of practices below may at first seem more like fun activities for sixth graders being introduced to human biology, because they are ways to see and do what may at first be grasped intellectually. But supplying memorized answers on a test demonstrates only one kind of learning. The kind of learning best suited for engaged practice of yoga therapy, from my point of view, concerns self-study that involves reflection and association rising from an embodied understanding. How someone feels in their state of disability is as important in this process as how someone thinks about it.

A major failing in western approaches to healthcare is termed "compliance." Patients don't comply, i.e., they don't do what they are told. Is this because they are patients and not participants in their own healing process? The system they seek help from inadvertently disempowers them from their own sense of agency.

As Porges writes,

In the Western world, we tend to place higher value on thoughts than on feelings. Parenting and educational strategies are targeted toward expanding and enhancing cognitive processes while inhibiting bodily feelings and impulses to move. The result is a cortico-centric orientation in which there is a top-down bias emphasizing mental processes and minimizing the bottom-up feeling emanating from our body. In many ways, our culture, including educational and religious institutions, has explicitly subjugated feelings of the body to the thought processes emanating from the brain. (2017, pp. 33–34)

How does this bias relate to compliance? Have you ever tried to lose weight, quit smoking, or begin an overzealous exercise plan? I once saw a *New Yorker* cartoon titled "The Mind-Body Problem," in which a person was sitting on the couch with a thought bubble of the mind saying "get up" and the body saying "no!" Motivation gets thrown around as the wedge to get the body to comply, but how does it work? Is it only the thoughts we say to ourselves in our heads, or does it require more than that? Does it require the feeling in the body of what a pain-free victory of being more fully abled would be like? From my experience of working with myself and others within the context of yoga therapy for the past 30-plus years, it is the body, the feeling state in the body, that brings about the change from within. The change in the feedback of the body provides what my teacher Aileen Crow called "the convincer." The felt reality of improvement spurs us on to to comply. This is not from the mind, or the reasons supplied, it is from the feeling state engendered and felt in the body that helps us turn the corner on reparations.

If this felt sense is needed, the more highly tuned the better. Tuning into one's anatomical geography can be learned and taught so that clients and patients learn to notice the effects of their patient practice. Not only that, but they also feel the importance of it. What does it feel like and what does the progress mean to them? As they move through their journey of healing they get back to the helm of their lives, more fully embodied, and ready for the adventure as it unfolds.

SOMATIZATIONS OF PHYSIOLOGICAL PROCESSES

The somatizations below offer a way to visualize, feel, see acted out, and participate in featured processes of the body. As a teaching tool they can make these processes more explicit for better understanding through sensing and hearing as well as through touch and movement. As a learning tool for comprehending basic anatomical and physiological processes these types of embodied explorations are fun and memorable. As ways to embody understanding, notice what they engender in you. After participating, what questions arise? What memories or concerns come to mind? What, in your understanding of these topics, has changed for you?

SOMATIC PRACTICE: Cellular and mechanical breathing

The term cellular breathing comes from the work of Bonnie Bainbridge Cohen (Cohen, 2018, ch. 5) and Body-Mind Centering®. This exploration invites you to become aware of this fundamental process in relation to the more familiar external aspect of mechanical respiration—the movement of air into and out of the lungs.

1. Lie comfortably on your back. You may want a small cushion under your knees or your head. Close your eyes. Notice the parts of your body that contact the floor—sense as well your connection to the earth. Allow your body to relax. Soften the muscles. Allow the weight of your body to yield or fall into the field of gravity. Allow the earth to hold you.

2. Feel the skin that envelops your entire body. Take a moment to notice your skin all around the perimeter of your body: between your fingers, down your back, around the openings, everywhere. Notice your skin: this organ of protection; this many-layered barrier of great sensitivity and intelligence.

3. Now bring your attention to the breath. Notice your breathing. Notice the movements that happen in the body as you breathe. Notice the movements where you are breathing the air in and out. Now notice the movements farther away from this direct process in your body. Become aware that your entire physical body is made up of many, many cells, like a

collective of individuals with many things in common, and many things unique about each one of them.

These cells are of different types, different tribes, but all are your body's cells. They are different tissues, different teams of cells working together for a common aim. And they are all breathing. All the cells of your body are breathing. Each and every one is taking in nutrients and oxygen, then burning the nutrients in the cellular fire, or *tejas* (combustion) to generate energy—heat and light. Then each cell expels the waste.

4. Now notice the air entering your nose, carrying oxygen down through the trachea, into the bronchi, into the bronchioles, and then to the alveoli. The alveoli are like tiny clusters of grapes on a stem. Notice the exhale, in which the carbon dioxide retraces the pathway out of the alveoli, through the bronchi, up through the trachea, and out of the nose and/or mouth. This is external respiration. Can you follow this pathway in for several breaths? Now switch your focus to following this pathway out for a few breaths. Now as you breathe, gently let your awareness rest on the flow of air in and out of the lungs.

5. Now go back to the feeling of the lungs and imagine the oxygen molecules crossing the single-celled walls of the alveoli into the bloodstream. Focus on this transition as you breathe for a few moments. After entering the blood, the oxygen gets a ride on the hemoglobin molecule and, on it, the oxygen flows through the blood to all the tissues of the body, to all the other tribes of cells. Take a moment and imagine this dispersion.

Then, each and every cell takes in the oxygen, and it arrives at the place where the cell has a little furnace, the mitochondria, where *tejas* or combustion happens. It is like each cell has a cellular furnace. And this is where the fuel from our consumption of food meets the oxygen within the flow of our air. Here is where our eating and our breathing match up and are transformed in our cellular fire. Energy now becomes useful to us, and we can use it to live. We live well if this process goes well and is balanced. The collective of cells that make up our body lives less well if this process does not go well or doesn't go well in specific areas or systems.

6. Take a moment and imagine the cells of your body using oxygen to burn the fuel you have taken in to create energy. Search your body for areas that are not as available to your perception, or where you notice less engagement in this fundamental life process. Cells themselves also exhale in a sense, in that they expel waste through their cell walls. This refuse goes back into the bloodstream and joins with other flows of excretion. In essence, then, through their cell walls, which are smart membranes, the cells are breathing. They are minutely expanding from their center, and they are minutely contracting toward their center. They are breathing by taking in nutrients and oxygen and then expelling waste.

7. Feel the whole body, alive and breathing on the cellular level. Notice any areas that seem to be doing this well, whatever that means to you just now. Are you aware of any areas in which this does not seem to be optimal? What happens if you focus there?

8. Then, when you are ready, again feel the mechanics of your external breathing, the air coming into the lungs and then going back out. Can you maintain awareness of both forms of respiration: cellular and external?

Bonnie Bainbridge Cohen (2012) proposes that every cell has its own sense of identity. A single-celled organism is a distinct functioning entity. It consumes, expels waste, reproduces, and moves about. It relates to its environment. It can be thought to have rudimentary consciousness as it makes decisions as to its continued existence as its capability allows.

In my work as a yoga therapist this translates to mean that each cell has awareness and purpose and possesses its own anatomical structure and functioning. It's when a cell is confused about these things that it can become vulnerable.

Auto-immunity seems like a result of cellular confusion. "Who I am and what is my purpose" are not so clear to these challenged cells. The Sanskrit term *svastha*, to be situated in one's own health, comes to mind. A cell that is self-possessed and aware of itself exhibits this quality. Cancer cells appear to have lost their sense of integrity and relationship to their identity as they've become vulnerable to outside influence.

Cellular breathing is an imperative context in all healing. Many yoga practices emphasize cellular breathing without necessarily calling it such.

SOMATIC PRACTICE: Digestion somatization

There are hosts of digestive conditions arising from varied known and unknown simple-to-complex causes. Diet, constitution, structural issues, impact of other diseases and medications, eating style, stress, gut flora, and even chewing all have an effect. Tuning into the digestive system anatomically can be a way for someone to begin to tune into their digestive function. This could lead to further examination of their manner of eating, eliminating, and assimilating what the world has to offer and the way that it does so. This somatization is not meant to be curative but is a simple starting point for orienting toward, understanding the location of, and embodying the digestive system and tract. It can be a meaningful experiential point of departure for further exploration.

INTRODUCTION TO THE DIGESTIVE SYSTEM AND PROCESS

The digestive system consists primarily of the gastrointestinal (GI) tract or alimentary canal along with the liver, gallbladder, and pancreas. The GI tract itself is one long hollow tube or series of organs from mouth to anus. My physiology teacher used to call it "the great outdoors" as it pretty much is the hole in the donut of our body. The parts of this inner tube are the mouth, esophagus, stomach, small intestine, large intestine, and anus. The liver, pancreas, and gallbladder are solid organs that support the breakdown of food during the digestive process.

SOMATIC PRACTICE: The path of digestion somatization

In this somatization we're going to follow the path of an item of food through the digestive tract (Figure 2.1) and, while doing so, I'll be sharing a few details about it as we go. You may sit, but I feel it would be best to lie on your back or side in a comfortable position. Feel free to move as you like or change positions as we go along.

Imagine taking a bite of some food you like

and that you know does well for your system. Notice any saliva in your mouth as you visualize and imagine taking into your mouth a desirable food item. You have three pairs of large salivary glands: the parotid glands in front of and just below your ears, the submandibular glands below the jaw, and the sublingual under your tongue. There are many smaller glands as well.

Chewing the food as needed and moving it around with the tongue, the food becomes more liquified, at which point you will swallow. Swallow and notice this action. If your mouth is dry and if you would like, take a sip of water to feel swallowing more effectively. To swallow, your tongue pushes food into your throat at which a small flap called the epiglottis folds over the windpipe or trachea to prevent choking. The epiglottis is located just behind the tongue and above the trachea. Take a moment and swallow a few times. Notice this action. With this, the food moves into the esophagus.

Use your hands to locate the area of your thorax that the esophagus passes through. Gently touch the area of your upper neck where the epiglottis is found. Then feel inside your body behind your trachea and in front of your spine to see if you can imagine and sense the location of the esophagus. Use your hands to sense this as well.

The esophagus is a hollow ring of muscle that runs from above your voice box to your stomach, which is in the left middle area of the upper abdomen. In adults the esophagus is usually between 10 and 13 inches long (25 to 33cm) so it's going to come down to where your ribs move out to the sides. It is about three-quarters of an inch (2cm) across at its smallest point. If you like, place your hands over this area. Perhaps do some movement to see if you can move with awareness of your esophagus.

Once something is swallowed the action of peristalsis becomes automatic. The layers of muscles in the esophagus and throughout the GI tract enable their walls to move. This wave-like movement pushes food and liquid through the tract as well as mixes the contents. Muscles trailing the food contract and squeeze, while the muscle ahead of the food relaxes. This allows the food to move downward.

At the ends of the esophagus there are specialized rings of muscles called sphincters. These function to stop flow into and out of this passageway. They are the upper esophageal sphincter, which relaxes to open the esophagus for food, and the lower esophageal sphincter, which controls the movement of food from the esophagus to the stomach. The lower usually remains closed to keep the stomach's contents from flowing back up into the esophagus. Swallow with the awareness that this closure will open. Then see if you can locate the juncture between the esophagus and the stomach. Notice what you notice there.

Now place your hands where you estimate your stomach is, which is to the middle left of your upper abdomen. See if you can get a sense of the size and dimensions of the stomach as you sense inside in this area. It is shaped like the letter "J" as if you were reading that facing yourself, i.e., the tip of the loop of the "J" is toward your midline. The stomach is a muscular mixing container for food, liquid, and digestive juices. Does your stomach have food in it or is it fairly empty? How do you know?

It takes anywhere from two to six hours for the stomach to empty, depending on the make-up of its contents and the psycho-emotional state of the individual. The semi-fluid mixture at this point is called chyme. It moves in a slow controlled way into the small intestine through a valve called the pyloric sphincter, located at the very bottom tip of the "J." Using your hands on your abdomen, see if you can locate and visualize your stomach. It can stretch and shrink depending on its contents.

Continuing the journey of digestion, see if you can gain a sense of the location of the pyloric valve as it empties into the small intestine. Similar to those in the rest of the tube, muscles of the small intestine mix the chyme with more digestive juices, which have entered the parade from the pancreas and liver, and push the mixture forward. The walls of the small intestine absorb water and digested nutrients into the bloodstream.

The small intestine lies coiled within the lower abdominal cavity and is framed by the large intestine. The small intestine has three parts. The first part, called the duodenum, is shortest, averaging about one foot (30cm) in length. The jejunum is second and runs about seven feet, while the ileum is even longer. It's around nine feet on average, and runs to its end at the ileocecal sphincter, which separates it from the large intestine. Place your hands over this area and imagine this long coiled-up tube within the pelvic and abdominal region. What do you notice when you do this?

The ileocecal valve is like a gateway about halfway between your hip bone and belly button that marks the start of your large intestine. The first part is called the cecum, which is a pouch-like structure, with the appendix, a worm-shaped tube, just below it. To locate the appendix there is a diagnostic point you can find called McBurney's Point. With your hands, locate the anterior superior iliac spine on the right side, then locate your navel. Roughly halfway between these two will be this point, which is over your appendix. The palpatory practice is to use your fingers and push into the abdomen and allow for rebound here. I'm including this only for informational purposes. You

may wish to simply locate this organ and sense its relation to the cecum and the ascending large intestine along that side of your lower abdomen.

The large intestine surrounds the small intestine like a square question mark, with the tail of the question mark ending at the anal canal. Its main job is to absorb water, which changes waste from liquid into stool. Peristalsis then moves the stool into the rectum where it is stored until you are ready to eliminate it through a bowel movement. The large intestine includes these parts: the appendix, the cecum that we just mentioned, the long tube of the colon, and the rectum, which is like the unloading dock at the end of this process.

With your hands, locate first the ascending colon on the right side of your lower abdomen, then cross from right to left around the level of your tenth ribs. This is the transverse part of your colon. Then find the descending colon traveling down the left side of your lower abdomen. The sigmoid or "s-shaped" segment goes from the lower left quadrant to your midline and is the little hook of the question-mark shape. This is the holding area for fecal matter, which moves then into the rectum—the antechamber of the unloading dock. The anus is the actual opening. Place your hands over the area of the location of the sigmoid colon and rectum. The anus is also a gateway or sphincter muscle.

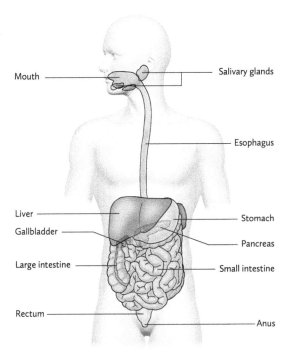

Mouth

Salivary glands

Esophagus

Liver

Stomach

Gallbladder

Pancreas

Large intestine

Small intestine

Rectum

Anus

Figure 2.1 The digestive tract

This somatization is the starting point of investigation. You could add the functions of each organ as well as mentioning the role of enzymes and other attributes of the digestive process if you like. In this example we kept to sensing and locating. This alone can be quite eye-opening to patients and clients who experience discomfort and who have had a disembodied relationship with their digestive tract. Somatic practices like these can help someone learn to be comfortable with what is inside of their body. They are then better able to comply with recommendations and practices for remediation of their difficulty.

A next step might be to lead a somatization with regard to how the hormones and nerves work together to help control the digestive process. The role and location of the vagal nerve is coming up in this chapter as well.

MOVING THE PATHWAYS

The body is a body of movement. Movement is not only a sign of life, it is fundamental to its processes. Understanding the body's processes can be done by moving them. Greater or lesser detail can be included depending on the topic and purpose. Think in terms of following a simple pathway through the body. Any pathway of movement of substance, electrical signal, hormones, and the like can be moved.

MOVING CIRCULATION THROUGH THE HEART AND BODY

Heart disease is the leading cause of death worldwide. So having a sense of where the heart resides and what it actually does can be a good orientation for those wishing to work with themselves. A somatic understanding, that is, a felt understanding, creates an intimacy along with embodiment. It connects us to our concerns and as I put forward above, encourages a better relationship with the health practices recommended by healthcare providers. It can help with our motivation to move, eat, and behave in healthier ways.

HEART ANATOMY BASICS: SETTING UP THE STEP-BY-STEP FLOW OF BLOOD THROUGH THE HEART

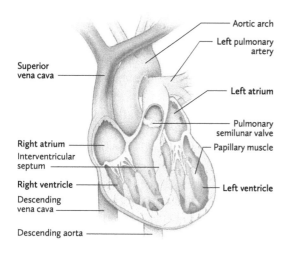

Figure 2.2 Cross-section of the heart

The heart is separated into two sides, right and left, by a central tissue generally called the septum (Figure 2.2). The right and left sides of the heart each have two chambers. Each has a smaller upper chamber and a larger lower one. The upper chambers are called the atria (singular is atrium) which, just like an entranceway to a building, are entry chambers. The lower chambers are called the ventricles, and these are more muscular, especially on the left side. A series of valves act like one-way doorways that control blood flow into and out of these four chambers. There is a valve from each atrium to each ventricle; these are generally called the atrioventricular valves. Then each ventricle also has a valve located more toward the middle of the heart going into a blood vessel.

SOMATIC PRACTICE: Moving circulation through the heart

Place your hand or hands over the heart, which is central and a little to the left under your sternum. Imagine, on your right side, two chambers, smaller on top and slightly larger and a tad longer on the bottom, with a one-way valve from top to bottom between them; this is the tricuspid valve. Next imagine, on the left, two chambers. One smaller on top has the same basic shape with a one-way valve from bottom to top between them. If you like, stop and draw this image for yourself.

Now continue by bringing awareness to the next set of valves. On the right side, more central than the tricuspid and a bit anterior, is the pulmonary valve. It is the one-way doorway between the right ventricle and the pulmonary artery, which takes deoxygenated blood to the lungs for refreshment. It leaves the ventricle on a vertical pathway then splits horizontally to each side toward each of the two lungs.

Return to the heart and find the left ventricle, the beefier lower chamber on the left side. Its second valve is also medial to its atrioventricular valve, and also is the one-way doorway to a blood vessel that ascends vertically out of the heart. This is the aortic valve, and it opens to the aorta, which is the first tube the blood enters after leaving the heart and before it is distributed throughout the body. The aorta ascends for about two inches (5cm) on average and then makes a beautiful arch and travels downward behind and a little left of the heart, having also branched into three vertical-traveling vessels at the arch's top.

The cardiac conduction system sends out electrical impulses that contract and relax the heart muscle. Those pulses set the rate and rhythm of your heartbeat, which sends the blood along its way. We'll explore the timing of this marvelous process a bit later; for now let's follow the pathway of the blood, and in slow motion, so we can follow along while visualizing and feeling what we feel. In this somatic practice we'll somatize the blood entering the heart, going to the lungs, returning to the heart, and then going out through the body. We're also going to move the hands to indicate some of the heart muscle activity and to better sense the action of the valves.

1. Please sit or lie down and use your hands over your heart as you like to sense what is happening.
2. Your heart is about the size of your own two hands clasped together and is central and a tad to the left under your breastbone or sternum. Find the right atrium in your imagination and locate the general area in your body as best as you can. Imagine the blood that has been circulating throughout your body entering this first chamber from above and below.
3. Now use your hand and gesture a gentle contraction as the right atrium contracts and the tricuspid valve opens and blood flows downward through this one-way door into the second chamber, the right ventricle. The valve closes and now the right ventricle contracts more powerfully. Use your hands to gesture this as you imagine the blood flow up and through the more central pulmonary valve. The one-way valve closes as the blood flows to both lungs. There the blood is reoxygenated. (See Somatic practice: Cellular and mechanical breathing.)
4. Spread the hands out over the lungs and sense the process of gas exchange. Now imagine the freshly oxygenated blood flowing back into the heart through the pulmonary veins off the left side of the left ventricle.

5. Gesture a tiny squeeze as the right atrium contracts, sending blood through the one-way door of the mitral valve into the left ventricle. This ventricle tends to be stronger as its job is to send the blood out to the whole body. Imagine this ventricle contract, squeeze the hand to indicate this, and imagine the one-way aortic valve opening and allowing the blood to move upward into the aorta and further upward toward the neck and head, and plunge downward and throughout the rest of the body.

Blood returns to the heart through the two large blood vessels called the superior vena cava and the inferior vena cava. They empty their deoxygenated blood into the right atrium and then the process begins again!

6. Now one more step, if you like. Take your impression of the pathway of blood into and through the heart and into the body and back to the heart, and use your hands to make a sort of dance that illustrates it. Think it though or say it out loud as you go, or even record the writing above and move to it as it is narrated. Then let go of the word, and let your arms and whole body, or however you like, move the pathway of blood as you recall it. Allow your movement to be big or small, in your whole body, or just your hands.

Now let go of the movement when you are ready. Notice how you feel. What do you notice? How does your heart feel? How is your circulation flowing? You may wish to note what you notice or share it with another person.

EMBODYING THE VAGUS NERVE

The autonomic nervous system keeps us in the game of life by responding to external and internal signals according to how we are patterned to perceive them. Neuroception, a term coined by Stephen Porges, describes the ways this system operates to detect threats and determine safety before and below our conscious awareness. Neuroception is foundational and acts as a platform, as Porges calls it a neural platform, on which our operating strategies for living are based. As we navigate our world, you could say our vagus nerve is part of our nervous system, "listening" to it. The vagus has a huge role in managing our states of being by regulating our body's key functions such as heart rate, blood flow, breathing, and digestion. It has a large role in helping us down-regulate to recover from stressful situations—real or imagined—at the physiological level. In doing so it helps us manage risk and orients us toward connection that will change our physiological and psychological state.

The vagus nerve is the tenth cranial nerve, which travels a long meandering path through the body from the medulla oblongata of the brainstem to the colon (Figure 2.3). The name, vagus, comes from the Latin *vagary*, meaning "wanderer," as in the word vagabond. It is the most influential nerve in the parasympathetic nervous system, having both afferent (sensory) and efferent (motor) fibers. Its importance is complex as it has many functions.

The upper portion of it carries sensory information about pain, touch, and temperature from the throat, regions of the inner and outer ear, and the meninges, or protective covering of the brain, near the back of the head. It also receives sensory information from the larynx, esophagus, and heart, has a minor role in taste, and carries sensory information from both baroreceptors and chemoreceptors in the aorta, which detect changes in blood pressure and sense oxygen levels in the blood respectively.

It has a critical motor role in speaking and swallowing, controlling movement of some of the muscles in the pharynx, larynx, and soft palate (and one muscle in the tongue).

As the main parasympathetic nerve of the body, moving into the chest and abdomen, it provides parasympathetic innervation to organs throughout the neck, thorax, and abdomen. To the heart, the right vagus nerve's cardiac branches mostly convey parasympathetic innervation to the sino-atrial (SA) node, while the left's branches mostly innervate the atrio-ventricular node (AV). These nodes reduce the resting heart rate, balancing its sympathetic activation.

In the abdomen the vagus nerve provides parasympathetic innervation to the bulk of abdominal organs with branches to the esophagus, stomach, and much of the intestinal tract to the splenic flexure of the large colon. Here the vagus nerve stimulates smooth muscle contraction and glandular secretions. For instance, in the stomach, the vagus nerve increases the rate of gastric emptying and stimulates acid production.

Through the actions of the vagus nerve, the parasympathetic nervous system is both our system of immobilization and our system of connection. The vagus is in fact not a single nerve but rather a bundle of nerve fibers woven together inside a sheath. A helpful image is an electrical cable that contains a number of wires inside its outer covering.

The vagus travels downward from the brainstem to the heart and stomach and upward to the face through its connection with other cranial nerves. The vagus is a mixed nerve, communicating bidirectionally between the body and the brain. Eighty percent of its fibers are sensory (afferent), sending information from the body to the brain, and 20 percent are motor (efferent), sending action information back from the brain to the body.

With 80 percent of its fibers bringing

information from various organs and muscles to the brain, a large part of what it does is check in with the heart, stomach, and the digestive tube and other organs. It relays this information to the housekeeping center of the brain, functioning below awareness. In terms of safety, we're also unconsciously scanning our environment for clues as well as noting subliminally the facial gestures and vocal tones of our compadres. We are hardwired to sense our internal and external environment for signs of threat and safety.

There is much talk about the vagus nerve and polyvagal theory, and work is being developed to establish safety and ease in the therapeutic encounter using what is known about the vagus for progress in therapy. It seems useful then to some degree to locate the pathway of the vagus generally in the body to grasp more fully and explore more deeply its impact in our work and in establishing safety connection, context, and choice.

SOMATIC PRACTICE: The vagus nerve

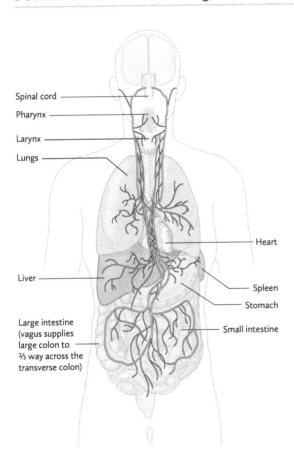

Figure 2.3 The vagus nerve

To imagine the vagus it can be helpful to imagine it not as a single strand but more as a bundle of

strands moving together within a sheath. If you've ever seen a group of electrical wires of different colors within a covering, this image is apropos. It's been called a conduit of connection because it interfaces not only with the brain and its target organs but also connects to other nerves like others going to the face and eyes. The vagus nerve is the most complicated of the cranial nerves because its functions are so widespread, innervating tissues in the neck, thorax, abdomen, and pelvic cavity.

1. Sit or lie down. Be comfortable. To trace the vagal pathway, as we travel along its path, you may wish to place a hand on your cheek and a hand over your heart. Then move one hand to your abdomen as you like. Experiment with moving your hands between these three positions as you imagine the vagal fibers connecting these physical locations.

2. The origin of the vagus nerve is in the medulla oblongata. The medulla oblongata is located at the bottom-most part of our brain. It helps control vital processes of heartbeat, breathing, and blood pressure. Sense within and notice this part of your head just below and a tad behind your ears.

3. The right and left vagus nerves exit the skull through the jugular foramen on each side of the foramen magnum. The foramen magnum is the passageway of the central nervous system through the occipital bone of the skull connecting the brain with the spinal cord. To locate this, feel the inferior aspect of the occipital bone as it approaches the atlas or first vertebra. Now palpate to the sides of your neck until you feel the lateral processes of your cervical spine. Your spinal cord will lie centrally between these two points. Imagine and feel the space upward between them and you will have the location of the foramen magnum. To each side of the foramen magnum are the occipital condyles, which protrude like tiny coffee table legs and fit into the atlas to begin the stack of the spine under the skull. Just lateral or outside to these on each side, and slightly anterior or forward, are the jugular foramen, which are created as an intersection between the medial temporal bones and the anterior lateral aspects of the occiput.

4. The jugular foramen is where the vagus passes out of the skull along with cranial nerves nine and eleven, as well as with the internal jugular vein. So as you sense and imagine there, see also the vein carrying blood from the brain as well as the other nerves. It is encased in the carotid sheath once it passes through this opening. The carotid passes into the skull through the carotid canal, another opening nearby.

5. Since the vagus has both sensory and motor pathways, for our purposes of location just allow yourself to sense and imagine connection and communication. Don't worry too much about direction. There is also a superior ganglion and an inferior one just inside and outside of the jugular foramen. These are slightly larger areas so, if you like, imagine a bulge at each location.

6. Starting at the top and moving downward, the vagus carries sensory input from the outer ear and middle ear, from some of the meninges or coverings of the brain. At the inferior ganglia, motor information is carried downward to lower portions of the body. We'll return to this; for now, some taste reception from the tongue and pharynx travels this path.

7. Also, motor fibers that work to constrict aspects of the pharynx of the throat run from the inferior ganglia and team up with those of other nerves to innervate swallowing. These work as well with another vagal branch and other nerves of the larynx. So, take a moment and swallow a few times. There is another branch that affects the voice as well, so, if you are inclined, allow yourself to make some vowel sounds. A simple "ah" will suffice. In the face, the vagus is known to interdigitate with muscles of facial expression, so you may explore this as well, but, for now, we'll continue down into the chest or thorax.

8. Traveling downward, the next area of interest is the pathway of the recurrent laryngeal nerves, which branch off the vagus near the aortic arch. The cane-like top of the aortic arch is at your midline just under the sternum and slightly lower than the clavicles. On the left, the nerve loops under the aortic arch and the left common carotid artery and makes its way up to the larynx. On the right, it loops under the right subclavian artery and does the same. These innervate the muscles of the larynx, with the exception of the cricothyroid muscle, giving them control in the opening, closing, and adjustment of the vocal cords. They also play a part in carrying sensory information of parts of the larynx, trachea, and esophagus. Locate

the aortic arch centrally below the line of your collar bones.

9. Around the area of the larynx is another branch of the vagus, which goes to the heart and is called the superior cervical cardiac branch. As the nerve travels downward, it branches off again to a recurrent nerve called the recurrent laryngeal nerve. This has a sub-branch that goes almost immediately to the thoracic cardiac nerve to the heart as well. They regulate the heart rate through both the SA (sinoatrial) and AV (atrioventricular) nodes. Place your hand over your heart as you might to salute the flag. Sense the rate and rhythm of your heartbeat.

10. After the recurrent laryngeal nerve, the vagus nerve continues down and gives off more branches to the lungs. The left vagus bronchial branch supplies the left lung, and the right bronchial branch of the vagus supplies the right lung. Move your hands to where you sense the bronchial tubes entering the lungs. The vagus helps control the amount of air passed into and out of the lungs.

11. The vagus nerve, both left and right, follows the esophagus as it penetrates the diaphragm. As the left and right vagus nerves do this they begin to interchange fibers. Some of the left vagus nerve fibers cross over to the right vagus nerve and some of the right vagus nerve fibers cross over the left vagus nerve. So locate the esophagus behind your heart and sense its descension through the opening of the diaphragm called the esophageal hiatus, into the abdominal cavity. As you do, imagine the fibers of the right and left beginning to interchange as well.

12. Once the right and left vagus nerves arrive in the abdominal cavity, they change names, becoming (1) the anterior vagal trunk and (2) the posterior vagal trunk.

The anterior descends along the anterior surface of the esophagus, while the posterior descends behind the esophagus. During early development in utero, the stomach rotates 90 degrees in a clockwise direction along its longitudinal axis. This rotation places the left vagus nerve along its anterior side and the right vagus nerve along its posterior side.

13. So the posterior vagal trunk is mostly fibers from the right vagus nerve with some from the left. And the anterior vagal trunk will mostly be the left vagus nerve with some fibers from the right. As they travel below the diaphragm, they form a plexus called the esophageal plexus.

Take a moment to place your hands over your stomach. Now imagine and feel the right vagus nerve coming through the esophageal hiatus and moving behind the stomach. This is now called the posterior vagal trunk. Then imagine and feel the left vagus nerve coming through the esophageal hiatus and to the front of the stomach. This is now called the anterior vagal trunk. Another branch comes off this truck to stimulate the liver parasympathetically, so it is called the hepatic branch. It will also help with GI function.

14. Past this area the anterior and posterior branch rejoin to create the celiac branch, which further down enlarges to become the celiac ganglion, which then forms a celiac plexus. This plexus gives rise to several other plexuses which serve individual structures with a large degree of complexity.

To find the center of this complexity in your body, we'll locate the celiac ganglia and slightly below it the celiac plexus. It lies anterior to the abdominal aorta, which is along your midline, at the level of the lower portion of your kidneys. Place your hand there and imagine this communication hub of parasympathetic activity (rest and digest). From here communication is aimed at these organs. The pervasiveness of the vagus fibers is reminiscent of Spanish Moss on trees. We'll simply focus on each organ, but have the sense of this multiplicity.

15. Locate each one as best you can and imagine the pathway of sensory information moving from each one through this intersection and to your low brain.
   • The spleen is off to your left flank above your waist at the level of your floating ribs.
   • Your kidneys are outside your peritoneum, about two finger-widths on each side of your spine halfway under your floating ribs.
   • Your adrenal glands (suprarenal glands) are located on top the kidneys.
   • Your stomach is to the left and below your sternum.
   • Your pancreas is to the left side, moving to your back behind the stomach.
   • Your liver (remembering that there is also innervation above from the hepatic branch as well) is just under your ribs on the right side.
   • The ovaries in women and testes in men, the ovaries at each side and slightly above the uterus.
   • The superior mesenteric plexus in the center of your body at the level of the lower half of the kidneys and in front of the abdominal aorta, traveling to your small intestine.
   • The cecum, the lower right side of pelvis, the ascending colon traveling up the right side of the pelvis and the transverse colon, traveling across from the right to left sides of the pelvis.

In the pelvis, pelvic nerves originating from the sacral region of the spinal cord give parasympathetic innervation to the bladder and the urethra as well as some communication with the penis, scrotum, uterus, and ovaries, although some contribution does come from the vagus nerve via the celiac plexus.

16. Now take a moment and feel in your body the various areas that we've connected through the vagal pathways. What do you notice? What would reception from these various tissues and organs collectively provide? When you are ready, stand and move around a bit. Notice what you notice. Use your senses to perceive the place you are in and notice your reactions to it, and your thoughts and how you are feeling just now. Recall the myriad, Spanish Moss-like threads of communication throughout your viscera. Notice your connection to yourself and to your environment.

Perhaps you'd like to take a moment to write down any observations and draw any impressions you may have, or simply continue to sense what this somatic understanding gives to you.

POLYVAGAL THEORY AND SOMATIZATION

In yoga therapy, as in related therapies, Stephen Porges' polyvagal theory has taken hold as an orientation to working with trauma and improvement of untenable, unproductive patterns of response to life, people, and events. The framework it provides gives credence to the immense value of yoga's traditional vocabulary of practice, which works directly with the autonomic system to establish balance within it, and further, to establish reliable pathways of behavior leading to physiological change toward recovery from the stress of challenging situations.

Many traditional yoga practices are designed to foster behavior and an orientation to living that systematically utilize tools for managing and regaining autonomic balance throughout one's day, week, and life. In terms of parasympathetic activation, which is on the rest and digest side of things, vagal tone is a term used to indicate the body's ability to return to a functionally relaxed state.

In the therapeutic context, polyvagal theory brings forward the reality that behavior is not fully under conscious control and that the body has its reasons for reacting the way it does. Because it is our nature to organize experience in the service of navigating our lives, what starts as a nonverbal state of physical orientation or bodily knowing becomes the basis for how we operate. And because we are meaning-making beings, what begins as the wordless experience of neuroception can drive the creation of a way of being and a story that shapes our lives.

The theory points to the role of the autonomic system as a surveillance system that monitors cues concerning safety or danger and even life threat from within our body, and in our environment, which includes, of course, other threats. As a risk-manager, the autonomic nervous system operates at the body level below our cognitive functioning. I liken this to the term *vasana* from the yoga tradition, as it implies imprints as organizing forces that create tendencies and dispositions. Without going too much into discussion of the various ways of using this Sanskrit term, I'm pointing out the notion "pre-thought" here: that of the set-up or predisposition for what will form into personality traits and behavioral tendencies.

Neuroception is the term Porges created for this process through which the autonomic system evaluates risk without necessarily involving cognitive awareness. The task is for the system to shift the autonomic state to optimize survival. This goes on beneath our conscious decision-making on the body level.

In the complacency of first-world living, in which many interactions take place online in the comfort of our living space with life-threat seeming far away, something relegated to entertainment story lines, attentive concern for survival may seem remote and like overkill. Getting in my car and driving to the supermarket to pick up something for dinner has scant minor risk. I could possibly get cut off in traffic or the store clerk, who's been on his feet all day, may snarl at me as I count out my change. But this is nothing like what our ancestors had to go through to ensure safe shelter and a meal *sans* Netflix. This system with the vagus nerve within it is an ancient one operating at several levels within us. It helps us survive by setting the tone for our body to navigate danger, protection, and comfort to preserve its all-important homeostasis. A related term previously mentioned is *svastha*. *Sva* means self and *stha* is situated, grounded, or anchored. Our autonomic system helps us remain anchored in a steady state of adaptability and well-health. It does this beneath and below awareness, orienting us toward optimal survival odds based on our evolutionary physiology, our personal history, and how our nervous system is patterned to respond to what it senses as a biological imperative.

Autonomic balance is commonly known to refer to the body's attempts to maintain homeostasis between the two antagonistic aspects of the autonomic nervous system: the sympathetic and the parasympathetic. This division is focused mainly on the motor pathways from the brain and spinal cord to the target organs of these systems. Polyvagal theory also includes the sensory pathways from the organs to the brain and brainstem, and the bidirectionality of communication also present in the autonomic system. The theory emphasizes the difference between two motor pathways that travel through the vagus nerve in that each pathway originates in a different area of the brainstem.

One pathway, called the dorsal vagal (from the dorsal motor nucleus), is unmyelinated and terminates in visceral organs below the diaphragm. The other (from the nucleus ambiguus) is myelinated and terminates on viscera above the diaphragm. With this division, the theory then outlines a hierarchy of three biological pathways of protective response. Not only this, the theory goes on to postulate that the autonomic system reacts to challenges in the reverse of its evolutionary history.

The three divisions of the autonomic system in polyvagal theory are:

1. the ventral vagal—parasympathetic
2. the sympathetic
3. the dorsal vagal—parasympathetic.

The dorsal vagal circuit is considered by Porges to be the oldest (500 million years old). Its response is centered on immobilization, such as in feigning death as it shuts the body down in response to life threat. The sympathetic system, next to evolve (400 million years old), activates the body to fight or flee, whichever provides the best opportunity for survival. The most recent circuit is called the ventral vagal (200 million years old). It involves using the face, voice, and other features of communication and involvement with others as a viable option for survival through social engagement. It is sometimes called the social engagement system in this model. Not only does this give us access to other beings, it allows us to return to a sense of safety and support through this contact; this is called co-regulation.

The key idea is that we are hardwired; genetically predisposed to seek safety and, until our autonomic system determines that we are safe, we will react unconsciously through the process of neuroception to our environment, and the cues we sense there, to secure our position.

Deb Dana, author of *The Polyvagal Theory in Therapy* (2018), offers a wealth of guidance for exploring this theory in response to the ups and downs of daily life. In one instance, she provides the image of a ladder showing each of the three autonomic states, with ventral vagal occupying the top third, sympathetic the middle third, and dorsal vagal at the bottom (pp. 56–57, p. 217). Below ventral vagal are shown the words safe and social, with sympathetic, mobilized and fight or flight, and with dorsal vagal, immobilized and collapse. The ladder is used as a way to gain autonomic awareness and facilitate movement between the states so as to not get stuck in less desirable ones. It can be helpful to track our state of being throughout the day. Many mindfulness practices help to do just this. The polyvagal piece introduced here is to relate our emotional and mental state to this automatic–autonomic prime directive of our body to adjust for what it senses as safe or unsafe.

SOMATIC PRACTICE: Somatic safety awareness exploration

Even without going to the level of life-threat and complete shut-down, as in fainting, we could study our body's felt sense in terms of safety, tracking whether we find ourselves ready to connect and engage socially, activate with our body upping its tone, or shut down, moving toward checking out, as posed by the polyvagal model. This is what I'd like you to do—track your experience in terms of the three items listed below.

For this exploration, choose an everyday activity, like going to the grocery store or running some other kind of errand. Have a clear beginning and ending to the exploration, and from start to finish keep track of your state of being in terms of these three states: social and safe, mobilized, and immobilized.

1. Social and safe: Do you feel a sense of ease in your body and are you open to having an encounter with other people and things you meet during your exercise? Will you say hello, chit chat, smile, make eye contact? Or do you feel that this, or a similar form of social connection, is not a possibility for you?

2. Mobilized: Do you feel reactive and/or activated in your body, like you wish to act somewhat aggressively, or you want to cut and run, like get out of Dodge pronto? This sense of aggression could be with words, like being rude to a salesclerk or the person in front of you.

3. Immobilized: Do you feel vacant or not really "in" your body, like it's offline in some way? Are you turned well inward and withdrawn from the environment? For your errand, do you do the actions but keep everything close to the chest, without taking in much or engaging with others, and having the very minimum interaction with things and people during your chore?

You may move between these states. From my experience of going to the market, I began pretty much at ease and connected to others, waving to a gentleman to cross the street while I smiled and waited at the stop sign. But then another driver at the busy road I needed to get on pulled right into the intersection and stopped, not allowing me to enter the line of traffic during my turn to go. I felt my body tighten as I raised my hands in the "What are you doing jerk?" gesture. When I got to the store, I noticed a bunch of teenage boys teasing a younger boy and it brought me back to my sixth-grade experience of being chased home by bullies about their age. It was during a snowstorm in which I ran out into the fields behind my house. I waited out there for hours until dark, so I could get home without being harmed. I was cold, wet, and exhausted, and my mother yelled at me for worrying her. At this remembrance, I felt my chest hollowed. I was no longer interested in shopping and wanted to disappear. Then, remembering that this was not happening to me, I activated, walking quickly to the customer service window. I smiled at the store manager as I said I thought some boys were ganging up on a much smaller boy in the candy aisle. I knew this manager was a dad, his son and my daughter had playdates when they were little, and he seemed like he could probably handle them.

In this example, I move from a safe and social mode to a defending and aggressive one, to moving toward shutdown. Then when I decide to act in the present moment, I mobilize and move toward a sort of forced social engagement where I talk to the manager whom I already know to be a "good guy." What happens for you during your exploration?

THE BIG IN AND THE BIG OUT (AND VICE VERSA)

Somatically speaking, for me, working to find ventral vagal, sympathetic, and dorsal vagal activation is most useful when I track my behavior in typical social settings. To me it feels like a global tracking of behavior, thought, and emotion during interaction with my world. I find it to be a useful practice to help me understand the role of my nervous system in setting me up for behavior that may be useful or not in settings in which I find myself. Exploring polyvagal theory in this way is using a mental construct that I must apply to the experience of my body. And the complexity of it to some degree takes me out of my embodied experience of myself, especially when the theory does not match my experience organically.

The question somatically (i.e., on the body level) of "how far in" I feel I am and "how far out" into the space around me and thus ready to engage with others in that area, is an investigation that I can more easily locate immediately in my body. Of course, "going out" and "coming in" in terms of nervous activity can directly relate to the sensory and motor nerves, some of which are autonomic. Is my intention to be sensing or motoring? Am I motoring to sense, or sensing to motor? Which is dominant in my experience? Am I doing both equally and how is what I'm doing supporting my intention, i.e., is it working well?

I was struck by the statement I heard that a cell cannot bond and defend at the same time. It is binary—a yes or a no. And this can relate to the sense of safety the autonomic system is busy assessing. Are we okay or not okay? Trustworthy, or not so? Human interactions are certainly more complex that a simple yes or no, and that fact holds great nuance.

Yet this idea of duality, of polar opposition, is one that the yoga tradition addresses in myriad ways. The tradition from which I draw utilizes the observation of nature and its features as tools for use in yoga practice. In a fundamental way, duality itself is credited for existence, one begetting two, and bursting forth into the multiplicity of form. Without duality, there is only union and no activity. Once two exist, there is a dynamic between them, an oscillation, an ebb and flow, that can be characterized as vibration—the essential feature of material existence. This is both spatial and temporal—existent things have a location in time. Fixing our point of view to one of the two items of a twosome, the experience

from that singular point of view is of self and not self, or self and other.

My experience of existing, then, is of traveling out from self and returning home. If I transition into space all around me instead of to only one point or direction in which I may go, I can experience a sense of enlargement or multidimensional expansion and then a return to a more singular point of smaller, reduced space. It is this experience, of expanding my awareness, my identity, and my movement by physically taking up and moving into more space, and then condensing and retreating to a smaller place that is "mine," that I call "The Big Out and the Big In." I mean it to be very comprehensive, in the way that Sanskrit words can have many shades of meaning and can be applied in myriad ways.

The vocabulary of yoga and Ayurveda uses the terms *brahmana* and *langhana* for the overall sense of expansion and reduction respectively. These terms commonly refer to the breath and to working with the expansion of inhalation and the emptying of exhalation. Interestingly, it is not only in this context that these terms refer to the sensation of expansion by filling the lungs and the condensing of emptying them. The terms also refer to the innervation of the sympathetic system on breathing in with the resultant increase of energy, and the parasympathetic activation of exhalation and subsequent sense of calm engendered.

A basic fetal rhythm develops in the early weeks of life that organizes various body parts into a whole-body experience. It can be seen in the flow of fluids from front to back and front again as the fetus develops, and later in the peristaltic waves of the digestive system that underlie a subtle alternating rhythm of flexion and extension.

These patterns together form a baseline rhythm of interchange that can be seen in all later movements and interaction patterns. The pattern can be experienced as one of in to out, and of going out to returning in. It includes all that happens and can be experienced along the way, such as being outward in some parts of oneself while inward in other parts or being stuck somewhere on the continuum unable to move in either direction. As a part of nature, our body also requires an attunement to this fundamental feature of existence.

Our autonomic nervous system holds such a subtle baseline of alternating rhythm. It helps us to manage when we must attend more to our environment or when we can simply be or flow with others in a context of connection and possible enjoyment. Also, there is always a rhythm of expansion and condensing going on in the body in general, and very specifically in many of the body's functions such as in breathing, the heartbeat, and the flow of cerebrospinal fluid.

Our attention and intention, as well as our ability to skillfully engage with our world, require a rhythmic exchange so that we can continue to function optimally. For us to be healthy, we do best when we exert and recuperate; when we have some excitement and enterprise, but also rest and return to the hearth of restoration. Health issues, learning issues, emotional imbalance, and general exhaustion in the adult population can be connected to this need for a rhythmic exchange from internal to external states of being by all living creatures. Learning to navigate ways to states that give us what we need in a rhythmic exchange throughout our day and lives is a very valuable aspect of what yoga therapy can offer.

SOMATIC PRACTICE: "The Big In and the Big Out"

This exploration is adapted from an in-class experience taught in one of our trainings, by Kimberly McKeever. It is one that begins in movement, so please give yourself the opportunity to do it in movement. You can sit, stand, or lie on your side. On your back or prone gives you less availability to movement. But once you have the idea, if you commit to moving and not giving in to the comfort of the floor, it will work that way too!

Even though this is a movement exploration, please keep your attention on your sense of comfort in the amount of space you are inhabiting with your body. The exploration's goal is for you to examine and explore your sense of comfort and safety through the range of expansion into the space around your body and reduction or return to a smaller sphere of movement or kinesphere.

You'll be moving from inward or medial rotation, flexion, and adduction to outward, or lateral rotation, extension, and abduction, and back. Do this slowly and gradually so you can track your level of comfort and safety as you go.

1. Begin sitting comfortably, standing, or side-lying. Notice what you notice in the moment.

2. Allow your body to condense and fold inward as if densifying into itself. Narrow, flex, adduct, medially rotate, and take up less space into a small, fully flexed, fetal position. Condense as much as you can or wish to within your body's ability and your comfort. Notice your response as you notice how this feels to you. Stay here as long as you wish.

3. Now allow your body to expand away from its felt sense of center in this fully densified position. This will likely cause you to widen, extend, abduct, laterally rotate, and generally take up more space. Expand as much as you can or wish to within your body's ability and your comfort. Notice your response to how this journey into space and expandedness feels to you. Stay here as long as you wish.

4. Now, begin to move toward the condensed state. Allow yourself to pause anywhere along the continuum. Only go

as far as you like. See where you are comfortable. What is this like? What does it remind you of? How does it feel? Travel to or toward the condensed state until you are satisfied with that sensation.

5. Now begin to move more toward the expanded state. Allow yourself to pause anywhere along the continuum. Only go out as far as you like. See where you are comfortable. What is this like? What does it remind you of? How does it feel?

6. Now move freely as you like between condensing and expanding. Allow yourself to change positions, or travel through space,

or rest at any point. Go at any speed. Notice what you notice.

7. Now find a position anywhere on this continuum of in-to-out and out-to-in that feels just right to you. How far out is perfectly comfortable to you just now? How far in? Is this a whole-body experience or are their parts of your body that wish to be farther in while others wish to be farther out? Does this remind you of anything? What is your experience of comfort? Familiarity? Unfamiliarity?

8. Rest when you are done exploring. Take time to transition out of the somatization.

Attention to "The Big Out and the Big In" gives body-centered information on the degree of comfort in opening to what is beyond ourselves and degree of comfort in returning to our own inner sensing. We may have acquired a multitude of skills in integrating going out and coming in simultaneously, or we may have only a few options in our experiential repertoire. We can also see a person's basic set point of autonomic activation and in doing so may gain evidence toward assessing their *dosha*, their baseline of physical, mental, and emotional activity and tissue health, and thereby needs in terms of practice.

Finding one's own rhythms of extending out and condensing in is a way to establish capability in relation to both gravity and space, and beyond that to external exposure and internal comfort. Understanding one's own patterns of condensing and expanding gives insight into one's overall tone or level of activation in general, and in specific relationships and environments. How much comfort do I find in going out? How much comfort do I find in returning in? What are my needs in relation to my own fluctuations in autonomic and physiological tone?

HEART RATE VARIABILITY

Heart rate variability (HRV), also called respiratory sinus arrhythmia, is the variation in time of the interval between heartbeats which is controlled by our autonomic nervous system. The variation in heart rate with breathing is considered a sign of good health. Heart rate variability is used to discern how well our body recovers from stress and is related to overall fitness. It can

be considered a metric of general resilience, of well-being; of our *svashta*.

As you know, stress typically activates our sympathetic system, raising not only heart rate, but also blood pressure and breathing rate. This is so we have the physical readiness and resources available to meet a threat head-on. When not endangered, our parasympathetic system should bring these functions to a comfortable resting rate. When our heart rate variability is low (i.e., not very variable) it usually means we are not readily bouncing back from stress with our autonomic system keeping us in a more vigilant state. Consistently low heart rate variability indicates our bodies are not adapting to or recovering from stress, well. Self-observation in other areas may also point to this. We may not be sleeping well or are feeling overworked and depleted. We may face overwhelming emotional upheaval, be stuck in a cycle of chronic pain, find we're getting sick a lot lately, generally feel out of sorts and the like.

High heart rate *variability* means our autonomic system is doing its job bringing us back to a more balanced resting state of recovery from stressful circumstances. People displaying high heart rate variability are adaptable. They are able to work hard and play hard, then resume calm. This is generally considered being resilient and more impervious to stress.

Heart rate variability is best measured by an ECG and more recently by tracking devices now on the market like the Apple Watch or the Oura Ring, designed expressly for this purpose. These devices can track the small changes in the intervals between consecutive heartbeats (called R-R intervals). Monitoring the beats of our hearts is also be a somatic practice most of us have done at some point, perhaps when checking pulse rate during a cardio workout. Taking your pulse rate is done by counting the number of beats per minute (or for 15 seconds and multiplying by four) at the temple, wrist, side of the neck, or ankle. Perception on HRV begins with this pulse monitoring but is different, as pulse rate only averages the number of beats per minute. With self-monitoring HRV, once we locate our pulse, we pay attention to the exactitude of our heartbeat's rhythm or lack thereof. We may be able to detect a slight increase in its rate during inhalation and a slight rate decrease during exhalation. Learning to check for one's own HRV is a reliable, non-invasive way to monitor our body's balance between parasympathetic and sympathetic activity.

SOMATIC PRACTICE: Heart rate variability

To get set up for this practice, I find it useful to find an exceedingly comfortable position. Lie down or sit comfortably and settle in to a quiet, inwardly focused state of being for the best results. I find this is best done upon awakening, before thinking too much about the day ahead, and definitely before you have caffeine on board. The end of the day, when you are transitioning to sleep, is also a good time, unless you have had alcohol, which may also skew your results.

1. Take at least a minute to just be. Notice your breath. Allow it to flow smoothly and easily.
2. Locate your pulse either at the inside of your wrist or at the side of your neck. Take a moment just to notice your pulse: its rate, its robustness or weakness, its quality.
3. Now return to the breath, becoming aware of your inhale separately from your exhale.
4. Next, add in awareness of your pulse. See if you can notice any change in your pulse rate; it may be very slight or inconsistent. You are looking specifically for it to increase a slight bit as you inhale and potentially decrease a slight bit as you exhale. It may not do this consistently. Notice what you notice.
5. Being in a comfortable position will help you to pay attention and to stay with this practice for a few minutes.

If you wish to check this regularly, I've found it useful to do so at about the same time each day under the same conditions.

TELLING THE ILLUSTRATED STORY

Although we may imagine somatic work to be a deeply focused felt experience with accompanying subtle movement, eyes closed, with complementary gentle breathing, it can also be a way to understand anatomy and physiological processes, bringing them off the page and into our life. There are many complex processes that can be shared this way: the HPA (hypothalamic-pituitary-adrenal) axis, the inflammatory response, the movement of food through the digestive system, and many more fascinating processes. In fact, just about any process may be highlighted and its salient features understood through the practice of illustrated storytelling, much in the way a children's book might tell the fable of a hero's journey.

We recommend this version of somatic work for getting the basic gist of a physiological process after being introduced to the basic anatomy of the area and grasping the process's main function. A main pedagogical feature of effective learning is deciding on the level of detail and depth needed by the student at any point. After studying and learning various aspects of anatomy and physiology through an assortment of types of institutions and programs, my experience has taught me that it is best learned in waves. Of course, cramming for a medical school exam will preclude this time-rich luxury. But yoga therapists, who may educate their clients about features of their body's functioning, will find that selecting choice features for client education is an important skill. The point is that we want the client to understand. So telling the story of a relevant physical process by introducing the players and putting them on stage can forge a relationship with the body that is not only personal and deep but also informed by knowledge that intertwines with their practices for betterment. For students and teachers, clients as well as practitioners, illustrating a simple or more complex study gives a lasting impression. And as someone takes a more complex understanding of anatomy and physiology in manageable waves, the total depth of care that results when it comes to working with an injury, illness, or preventative program will be far more engaging and enjoyable than any complicated cram session would have rendered.

SOMATIC PRACTICE: Telling the illustrated story

For this practice we invite you to spend time studying a process of interest, either one of the above, or something else you have reason to be curious about—that makes it more meaningful and dare I say—fun! Then break it down into these features:

1. What is the function or purpose of this process generally speaking?
2. Where is the location of the process in the body?
3. Give a short synopsis. This helps the listener tune in by giving them an overview. It also gives the storyteller a sense of the listener's interest and ability to follow along!
4. Draw, or create a living diagram for moving through, or schemata to illustrate the process pictorially if at all possible.
5. Tell the story in simple terms from beginning to end.

There are two ways to do this. One writing out your tale or simply getting the story down in your memory so you can tell it, like a fairy tale or family story you may have told one too many times before. If you write it out, you can hand that information to your client. You can also do both! Which is a great feat, as you'll have created great handout materials for clients as well as having mastered (and by mastered, I mean have committed to memory) some important anatomy and physiology you can then build on and deepen into.

The other is drawing a diagram ahead of time and walking your client through it as you talk, or drawing while you're telling the story. This is rather like singing and playing the guitar. Doing both at the same time takes some skill. Some people can do both at the same time while others need to do one at a time. For the sake of articulating steps here, I've separated this drawing out into a different step.

It's fine to pepper your telling with facts you find interesting if you like. This not only makes the storytelling more robust, it can share your authentic sense of wonder in the body and of what it is capable. But, at least the first time through, try not to get too detailed or take too many side trips, especially into chemistry or details of pressure gradients and the like. Many people don't have that in their background and so you may lose them. And the value of fostering an interest in someone's own anatomy and physiology for the sheer health benefits possible is far too great. Please keep it as simple and straightforward as you can—even though the more you know about the marvel of the body's processes, the more exciting it is to share!

When you're ready, share your story with someone else or a small group of worthy learners. As you share, you can illustrate the tale by drawing on a large white board, or if online, sharing your screen while you draw. We use the Notability app for drawing, but Zoom and others now have a whiteboard feature. If you are in-person, please give creating an environment to enact the process in actual space a try! Make it a floor diagram and have your learner(s) move through it. If you have a driveway or parking lot you can draw the pathway with chalk, making it large enough for someone to move along the pathway. You can make a border using rope or yarn or even pieces of paper along the floor. Use office furniture or whatever you've got to represent the different features of the body and then have your learners, which could be your clients, move along the pathway or tour the structures you have created. It is infinitely more memorable and fun and brings the experience of anatomy to a lived and felt level of understanding. Imagine peering into the slender cattle pen of the ureter filled with the large physio balls as you work to understand the real possibility of a kidney stone developing in your own body. Then sense the pathway in your own torso that it would take. Memorable right?

Hearing the story told simply while walking through the process is reminiscent of the Isaac Asimov book and subsequent 1966 movie, *Fantastic Voyage*, in which a submarine of scientists shrinks to the size of a blood cell and journeys through the body to the brain. It is one thing to hear that you must clean up your diet; it is quite another to see the reasons for doing so lived large in Technicolor.

Here is an example of the features outlined above. We do this somatic practice in class from time to time about subjects that students may wish to be able to explain to their clients. It's a good learning tool, a good skill to have, and a good way to check on one's own understanding. For this example, I've chosen what several who have spent their lives studying the body have told me they understand to be one of the body's most elegant processes by one of its smartest organs—urine formation in the kidney.

1. What is the function or purpose of this process, generally speaking?

The kidneys filter the blood and produce urine. They remove waste and control the body's fluid balance, maintaining the right levels of electrolytes. Fun facts: All of your body's blood passes through them 40 or so times a day. And around 180 liters of blood are filtered by the kidneys every day.

2. Where is the location of the process in the body?

Ruling out anomalies, the kidneys are located a few finger-widths on each side of the spine, tucked under the bottom of, and below the lower ribs. They are retroperitoneal, which means they lie behind the membrane that surrounds the abdominal cavity that holds the intestines and stomach. They are actually shaped like the bean of their name and are about the size of that person's fist. The really cool structure in the kidney responsible for filtering the blood is called the nephron and has two main parts (which have subparts): the renal corpuscle and the attached tubular. Each kidney is going to have around one million nephrons in it!

3. Give a short synopsis.

Blood comes into the kidney, waste gets removed, and salt, water, and minerals are adjusted as needed. The filtered blood goes back into the body. Waste gets turned into urine, which collects in the kidney's pelvis—a funnel-shaped structure that drains down a tube called the ureter to the bladder and out of the body through the urethra.

4. Draw, or create a living diagram for moving through or schemata to illustrate the process pictorially.

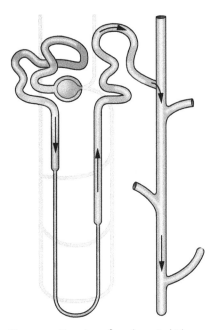

Figure 2.4 Drawing of nephron in kidney

5. Tell the story in simple terms from beginning to end.

The nephron is the main functional feature (Figure 2.4). It is a tube-like structure. On one end it's got a catcher's mitt cup called Bowman's capsule. This capsule encloses a ball-like cluster of blood vessels called the glomerulus, which in Latin means ball of yarn, because that is what it looks like. Its shape greatly increases the surface area for filtration. The first step of urine formation is where this tuft of vessels meets the Bowman's capsule. So picture a ball of yarn as the blood vessels and a cup surrounding it as the beginning of the nephron or filtration tube, or, better yet, make a claw hand with one hand, and then a fist with the other and place it inside the claw: you've got the glomerulus in the Bowman's capsule. The blood vessel that brings blood inside the glomerulus is the afferent vessel, while the blood vessel that takes the blood out of the glomerulus is the efferent vessel. We'll get back to this in a moment.

The Bowman's capsule is one end of a long tube that, at its beginning and end, is shaped like a silly straw end. If you've never seen a silly straw, this is to say that at either end the tube zigs and zags in convoluted folds. At the far end, after the second silly straw end, the tube, called the renal tubule, ends up in the duct system of the kidney. Before that is where the magic happens in the nephron. Between the two silly straw ends (the first part is called the proximal convoluted tube or PVT, and the last part is the distal convoluted tube or DVT) is a hairpin dip, looking a bit like the loop of a paper clip, called the Loop of Henle.

Along the entire length of the nephron is a network of capillaries that bring in impure blood, containing lots of waste products, and take out purified blood that has gotten filtered by the nephron. The blood enters the kidney via the large renal artery that branches off the abdominal aorta. After entering the kidney, the artery divides many times until the smallest one enters a nephron, bringing blood into the glomerulus. At the intersection of the glomerulus and the Bowman's capsule the first act of filtration happens. The filtration produces filtrate that goes into the nephron tubule as well as impure plasma that retains aspects of the blood, like blood cells and proteins, and this continues along its path in the efferent blood vessel.

The filtrate, that's what it's now called, next moves into the renal tubules where it is further processed to form urine. It needs further processing because it contains a lot of things that shouldn't be excreted as waste! This would be like throwing the baby out with the bathwater. There's a whole world of detail here on what happens and how, but in short, the descending tube (PCT), the hairpin curve (Loop of Henle), and the ascending tube (DCT) are like truck stops offering different services on a cross-country drive. Each place has a job to do in terms of reabsorbing things the body has decided it needs back in the blood. Because we don't want to lose valuable nutrients, water, salts, and whatnot, reabsorption takes place along the length of the renal tubule. Remember that the tubule is surrounded with blood vessels, which are called the peritubular capillaries. So it is through these that whatever gets reabsorbed is then passed back into blood circulation.

In the last part of the tubule, the DCT or ending part of the paper clip after the turn, the final mechanism of urine formation takes place. Here the walls of the tubule actively remove any lingering waste that escaped filtration. This waste combines with the remaining filtrate and becomes urine. It then flows into a collecting duct. The urine in each of the kidney's collecting ducts drain into the renal pelvis which in turn connects to the ureters. The urine produced then makes its way out of the body through the ureters to the urinary bladder and the urethra.

ILLUSTRATING THE STORY TO EMBODY ITS ANATOMY

While it is helpful to act out a physiological process with players in time, like a scene from a play, it can also be useful to illustrate anatomy in a large-as-life way. For yoga students and enthusiasts, many of whom are women of childbearing age, the pelvic floor and perineum are of particular interest. Here are two helpful ways to introduce the anatomy of the pelvic floor and perineum and sense the space, form, and muscles of this body area.

SOMATIC PRACTICE: "Draw with me" perineum

Another way to learn anatomical material and explore it somatically is to draw each element.

You'll need a piece of blank paper and some colored pencils or pens, and a few good anatomical images of the pelvic diaphragm and the perineum.

1. First sit on the center of the paper. With a pencil make a mark on it just underneath these four bony landmarks: (A) the coccyx under your tailbone, (B and C) both ischial tuberosities, and (D) your pubic synthesis.
2. Take the paper out from under you and draw a thin line connecting the dots.
    These will be your:
- sacrotuberous ligament from the coccyx/sacral area to your ischial tuberosities on both sides in the back
- ischiopubic rami, one on each side (ramus is singular), from the ischial tuberosities to your pubic symphysis.

You may notice this frame seems to be a different size than you expected, seems lopsided, or something else. Just notice your response. We'll use this as the basis of our drawing.

Before going on to drawing the muscles at the base of the pelvis, take a moment and to find these four borders. If you are comfortable and can reach, palpate each border, noticing what comes into view more easily and what is less available to perception. Also walk, dance, or do some standing poses or other actions while keeping in mind the lines from the coccyx to the tuberosities, then the lines from the pubis to them. What do you notice?

If you have an anatomy phone app or a *Netter Atlas of Human Anatomy* refer to these, or just look up some images of the muscles of the perineum. This will help you locate and see the dimensions and pathways of these muscles and structures. Finding one or more source images will be helpful. When we do this in class, the teacher draws the anatomy one part at a time on the board and participants then draw along with them. For the sake of simplicity, we'll draw a female pelvis. You can adapt this to the male pelvic source images if you prefer.

1. First draw four small circles down the midline: one close to the pubis as this will be the clitoris, the second a small bit posterior to it—this will be the urethra—and again a little behind that, a slightly larger circle for the vagina. These should be roughly in the anterior half of the diamond outline. Then add one more circle for the anus about a third of the way in from the posterior tip representing the coccyx.

    We'll begin drawing the muscles of the perineum from an inferior view. That means it is as if we are looking upward: as if you were lying on the floor, and someone stood over you—you would then have an inferior view as you are viewing from below. The perineum is bordered by the structures we identified above. Below it is skin, some fat, and fascia. Above it is the pelvic diaphragm. The perineum is commonly divided into two groups of tissues called the urogenital triangle and the anal triangle. The urogenital triangle contains the penis and scrotum in the male and the clitoris, urethra, and vagina in the female, and related structures.

2. We'll now add an important structure called the perineal body. Draw a small triangle or pyramid between the anterior portion of the ischial tuberosities for female anatomy or place it slightly anterior of the tuberosities for male anatomy. This connective tissue structure rises into the pelvic cavity with multiple layers of tissues using it as a support. I liken to this the physical sheath manifestation of the

svayambhu linga, around which Kundalini Shakti is wrapped three and one-half times, when she is in her dormant state.

3. Now draw two lines, one from each side of the perineal body to each of the ischial tuberosities. Take a look at the image you've selected as source image(s), then draw in the muscles in the color of your choice. These are the superficial transverse perineal muscles. Notice their line of pull. See if you can activate them on both sides of your perineal body. What do you find? What support do they give?

4. Next, we'll draw the ischiocavernosus muscles on each side. Draw a line from the medial aspect of the ischial tuberosities to the medial pubic rami on each side, leaving some space at the border between them.

5. Beginning at the pubic rami just between the ischiocavernosus muscle on one side, draw a loop that travels posterior and around the vagina and back to the other side of the pubis. This is the bulbospongiosus muscle. Check your source image and fill it in.

6. Next, we'll draw the levator ani muscles as one unit. We'll separate the parts of it in the next section. It is considered part of the perineum and part of the pelvic floor or pelvic diaphragm. The various names for these areas and the differences in the male and female anatomy can add confusion here. From our established inferior view, we'll only be able to see the posterior portion of this group of muscles. As the largest component of the pelvic floor, its muscular sheet attaches to the pubic bone anteriorly, the ischial spines, which run along the bottom of the ischial bones from your tail to your sit bones (due to early trauma, it took me years to find them), and to a thickened fascia of the obturator internus muscle. It's interesting to note that not all muscles travel from bone to bone, as some attach to connective tissues as well.

7. Finally, we'll draw the external sphincter ani muscles that ring the anus. It is secured in place by its connection to the perineal body anteriorly and by a ligament to the coccyx posteriorly.

SOMATIC PRACTICE: "Draw with me" pelvic diaphragm

You can layer these muscles on top of the ones you've drawn previously, but I prefer taking another blank sheet of paper, placing it on top of the drawing you've made, and outlining as best you can the diamond shape with the circles and triangle. From this we'll draw the next superior layer. Remember we are going from the very bottom of the torso upward.

Two muscles comprise the pelvic diaphragm, also called the pelvic floor. They are the levator ani and the coccygeus. The levator ani arises from each side of the pubic bone, fans out along the ischial spine, drooping a bit like a hammock as it crosses the pelvic outlet, and inserts on the coccyx and anococcygeal ligament. It has essentially four parts.

1. First, we'll draw the levator vaginae (in males this would be called the levator prostatae) from the most medial part of one pubic ramus, loop it around the urethra's hiatus (i.e., the circle you've drawn closest to the pubic bone), and return to the other most medial part of the other pubic ramus.

2. We're going to do the same basic thing for the next muscle, called the puborectalis,

except it will loop the opening to the rectum and begin and return just lateral to or outside the last muscle above, the levator vaginae.

3. Next is the pubococcygeus. As its name implies, this muscle will begin just lateral to the one you've just drawn on each side and travel outside both of these prior muscles all the way to the back of the pelvis, and attach onto the coccyx. In the middle of this is a midline raft of ligamentous tissue where the two halves of the muscles attach.

4. The fourth is the iliococcygeus muscle. It is even more lateral as it arises from the ischial spine and pelvic fascia and attaches to the coccyx and anococcygeal raft. Together these make up the levator ani.

5. On the same plane as the above muscles is the coccygeus. A triangular-shaped sheet, it originates from the ischial spine and inserts onto the lateral aspect of the coccyx and the sacrum along the sacrospinous ligament. The coccygeus together with the levator ani form the pelvic diaphragm.

SOMATIC PRACTICE: "Draw with me" general pelvic floor

Sometimes the front portion of this area, or in this case the front half of your diamond drawing, is called the urogenital triangle, while the back half is called the anal triangle. If you are one who has done a great deal of root lock, *agni sara*, or similar practice, it may well be fairly easy for you to isolate and initiate movement from each of these muscle groups. For many people new to yoga, this may not be the case. Also, sexual abuse and trauma can cause us to withdraw from areas of our body. Skillful, sensitive, somatically based yoga practice can help us reinhabit areas that has been traumatized. The somatic practice that follows this "Draw with me" exploration is an excellent place to introduce working gently and generally with this area.

A good starting point for locating, releasing, activating, and gaining good motor control over the muscles in this area is to begin working with imagery focusing on areas of the diamond shape you've just drawn.

1. Lie on your back with some support under your head and upper back, and locate your breath.

2. Begin by noticing any difference in tone of your pelvic diaphragm as you breathe.

3. Recall the diamond outline of the pelvic outlet with the coccyx the back tip, the two ischial tuberosities at the sides, and the pubic symphysis in the front.

4. See if you can sense a line of connection between the front tip and the back tip. Imagine a canoe shape from the coccyx to the pubis. As you breathe out, see if you can shorten the canoe. As you breathe in, allow it to return to a longer size.

5. Next sense the space between the two sides of the diamond, the ischial tuberosities. Draw an imaginary line between them. There are actually two layers of muscle here, as well as lateral connective tissue running laterally along this path. We only drew the superficial transverse perineal muscles, but there is a deep layer as well. And the perineal membrane can create a lateral line of force too. Explore doing the same as above with the breath: narrow from side to side as you exhale and allow for widening between the tuberosities as you inhale.

6. Next imagine dividing the diamond into four quadrants like one of those folded paper fortune teller games. See if you can activate or tighten only one side of the diamond or two squares at a time. Try the other side, the front only, then the back only. Play with other possibilities and combinations.

7. Another image that lends itself well to this body area is the fan-like shape that the muscles of the levator ani make.

Once you've envisioned the anatomy of this area to your satisfaction, stand and walk around. Notice what you notice. Take some time to integrate what you've explored.

MAKING ART AND USING FOUND OBJECTS

Draw what you experience to be a part or function of your body. Make a cartoon of your current understanding and questions. Build a model and then another one.

Illustrating the anatomy or physiology to learn where you're foggy on the exactness of a location or connection between parts will keep your learning connected to your source of creativity and curiosity. Rather than a dried-up chore, studying the body will be a lived, joyful endeavor. In your daily life, keep an eye open for found objects that give you an impressionistic sense of the body's structure or function. Notice or even create simple machines that demonstrate natural principles like fluid moving from higher pressure in the heart to lower pressure. Allow your life to be enriched by ways to deepen into your experience of this fleeting corporality.

Here are some things I've enjoyed discovering that relate to my study of anatomy and physiology.

- comparing the lines of the palms of the hand with the veins of a leaf
- winter tree branches looking like blood vessels
- bunches of grapes looking like the bronchioles and alveoli of the lungs
- grasses and flora on the earth resembling hair on the body
- weather system movements looking like swirls of body hair
- cargo netting behaving like fascia
- levers—seeing them helps me understand moving!

This may seem to you like too juvenile an approach. If so, I invite you to look at that judgment and ask, when did the playfulness of youth leave your life bereft of discovery?

SOMATIC PRACTICE FOR IMPROVING MOVEMENT EFFICIENCY

We move in relationship with all levels or our being and within the context of our environment. Movement efficiency then is not only about the "mechanics"; it requires the art and skill of being open, responsive, and adaptive. As a function of praxis, movement efficiency involves planning what to do, how to do it, and continually making appropriate adjustments toward completing a desired goal or action. Our experiences also pattern our future responses as we allow ourselves to be present to the ever changing moments.

Lauree Wise MSOT, CMA, Body Mind Centering® Practitioner

INTRODUCTION: EXPERIENTIAL FRAMEWORKS FOR OPTIMIZING MOVEMENT FUNCTION

Working toward greater movement efficiency is a large part of yoga therapy practice. Persistent pain and injury arising from misalignments, faulty body use, and other sources is an area of repatterning with which yoga therapists likely have personal as well as professional experience. A skillful yoga posture and *vinyasa* practice done over time with awareness can improve alignment and strip away extraneous muscle action and faulty use of the body as the practitioner learns to tune in and refine their technique.

Beyond the basics of knowing which part of the body goes where, contemporary styles of yoga often have detailed instructions on how to remain in the pose with push points, energetic imagery, and specific anatomical instructions like pulling up the kneecaps, or squeezing or releasing the gluteal muscles. Some systems focus on helping an individual remain steady in a pose. For our purposes, we are concerned with movement and, specifically, with moving efficiently. Most "mere mortals" coming to yoga therapy for a physical concern wish to get out of pain and stay that way. This involves moving in a way that will not continue to damage tissue, and thus part of our job is to teach movement efficiency. So while some yoga alignment techniques are very helpful, say when applying them to sitting well for long hours at a desk, they may not be enough where functional *movement* is concerned.

As yoga therapists, conveying just exactly how we want our clients and students to do a certain practice can be challenging. Especially where movement is concerned, we may find ourselves using a host of creative ways to express what we see in our students' movement and body use versus what we want to be seeing! Saying or showing verbally, using touch, and using demonstration are ways in which we seek to make these corrections. The yoga postures and *vinyasa* movements and their adaptations must be applied correctly with right activation for the therapeutic effect to be obtained.

As I've worked with people presenting with various physical issues over the past 30 years, I have noticed divisions in what needed to be addressed first, second, third, and so forth, depending on level of movement ability. Over time, I devised a framework for working with movement efficiency I call the Three Streams of Functional Movement Rehabilitation™. I see the streams flowing together the way rivers join in a confluence and then separate, only to rejoin further downstream with the waters joining and rejoining the others.

In this confluence of care, the three streams flow from dysfunction to optimal function for that person. An injured client on the mends may begin in the first stream and then progress through the other two streams, each time making greater improvement in their functional movement efficiency. Or a client beginning in a different stream may be assessed to need work in another stream, as each person is individual in their needs, and setbacks and side trips are a part of the trail to reclamation.

The streams may intertwine or remain separate. The first stream, Stream A, deals with specific trauma and injury recovery. Certainly acute injury is outside our scope, but the long, sometimes winding, road of recovery when addressed as an issue of movement efficiency can be worked with when carefully administered while tissues heal.

The second stream, Stream B, picks up on the progress made by getting out of a more acute state, and moves the client toward further refinement, from local use of the affected body part or areas, and to global use, reintegrating the injured part into the whole. This stream also functions well in addressing chronic dysfunction and pain, i.e., injuries that never made their way to pain-free full recovery for whatever reason.

The third stream, Stream C, focuses on improving movement skill. Sometimes there need not be any injury or pain. Someone may wish to learn how to perform better. This could be anything from learning how to do a pose like Crow (*Bakasana*) or Headstand (*Shrishasana*), to pedaling a road bike with less effort, to pitching a baseball with greater accuracy. Of course, movement skill is improved as part of any of the three streams and it is for this reason I call this model a confluence. I've found it useful in its ability to tailor the sequence of practices according to the precise needs and progression of the client. As we know, even two people with the same injury will progress at their own rate depending on a number of factors. In the realm of movement efficiency, already highly skilled movers can rely on their adeptness, while others may need to learn new ways of using their bodies.

FUNCTIONAL MOVEMENT REHABILITATION™

Functional Movement Rehabilitation™ (FMR) is an approach to move the client from injury or impairment to optimal movement function, whether for sports, dance, work, or daily life activity. The purpose of FMR is to retrain functional movement patterns toward optimal functioning. Functional movement patterns require that all the muscles and joints of the body work together in a coordinated manner. As dysfunction develops in one region, it may affect other regions, resulting in further problems and the spread of pain. Functional Movement Rehabilitation helps re-establish balanced myofascial co-activation and coordination in areas of injury or impairment and subsequently throughout the body. This helps individuals return to sports, dance, work, and other activities of daily life.

This work primarily involves the *anna maya kosha* (food sheath). Attention is chiefly on the skeletal bones and joints, along with the integrative use of the muscular, fascial, and nervous systems. Secondarily, working with organs, deep fascia, personal habits, body image, and deeper *koshic* levels may be necessary as well. But here we'll stay at the body level.

We lose movement function through:

1. *Trauma*: Acute injury can produce chronic compensation patterns of misuse; surgeries alter motor control and instigate muscular inhibition; other forms of trauma create holding and misuse patterns.

2. *Learned behavior*: Body image beliefs, inefficient physical training (bad ballet technique, bad piano technique, faulty tennis swing), hunched over, unsupported work and study postures combined with overwork and lack of movement, persistent trauma responses.

3. *Poor neurodevelopmental patterning*: Less than optimal opportunity to lead a rich and varied movement life from birth onward can result in poor neuromuscular organization.

Virtually every condition of chronic pain, less than optimal body use, and myofascial or skeletal injury involves some form of movement dysfunction and muscular inhibition. Synergists in a movement are the muscles that stabilize a joint around which movement is occurring. This in turn helps the agonist (prime mover) function effectively. With injury there is a trauma response in which the nervous system up-regulates the functional synergists to protect and stabilize the joint or area of concern. As the body up-regulates to support local or global instability, gripping patterns can result. Gripping patterns can become the cause in chronic "bad" (misaligned, inefficiently initiated and sequenced) postural and movement habits. These more global patterns are an attempt to compensate for muscle inhibition, weakness, connective tissue buildup, and other dysfunction. Common gripping patterns can be seen at the shoulders, hips, toes, and gluteal area. Propping patterns can also become the chronic "go to" pattern, especially due to weakness and easy muscle fatigue after long-term injury or one-sided movement. Propping is stabilizing in a position without sufficient motor control. Locked knees and elbows are common signs of propping. When we observe gripping or propping patterns, we should look to other related areas of the body in the performance of a movement to ascertain where the primary dysfunction lies.

Other substitution patterns, like increased overall tension, for instance, are used to meet movement challenges that are beyond someone's functional capacity. If used often, they become the norm. Like water always flowing to the lower point, the body will use patterns it has found that are easy. Then, due to regular use of these patterns of inefficient motor sequencing, a cascading effect of imbalance often takes place.

As a result, clients often present with several layers of dysfunction and multiple compensatory strategies and substitution patterns in place. The goal is then to determine the seed kernel of the client's dysfunction. The mystery to solve is: What is the greatest dysfunction responsible for the client's issue? While there can be several causes, one is likely to be primary.

Secondary ones are likely to be compensatory. The job then is to peel back the layers, and repattern alignment and movement efficiency for optimal efficient, effective, and expressive functioning.

This section will share several areas of somatic practice that promote improved movement efficiency. We'll visit featured areas of body use that together provide a comprehensive view of betterment of movement efficiency. We'll sample ideokinesis, or using visual imagery and the body's felt sense, to support skeletal and dynamic alignment. Then we'll explore how correct use of space in observing and practicing movement can provide clarity, articulation, and correct organization and sequencing of body parts and areas in movement. Crucial to refining movement efficiency, we'll explore somatic practices that provide much in the way of this sort of awareness for cultivating movement skill. Then we'll see how the quality of the movement, that is the movement's dynamics, can have a positive effect not only on bodily ease, but on the tissues performing the actions themselves.

CHAPTER 3

Embodying Static and Dynamic Alignment

Static alignment refers to alignment when the body remains in a position in space. Most work with alignment begins here with standing. Mountain Pose (*Tadasana*), sometimes referred to as Simple Standing Pose, is a posture in which a skilled observer can see much of the body use and whatever mobility, stability, strength, weakness, and body use patterning may be present in trace amounts. It is often the simplest things are the most revelatory!

Sitting posture, a very important posture in yoga meditation, needs to be as efficient as possible because in essence we want the body and its multifarious sensations out of the way so we can attend to the itinerant activities of mind to focus its attention. Many yoga teachers in trying to get their positional directions across use imagery and the imagination in concert with the students' felt sense and awareness of their body. In fact, in many systems of somatic learning awareness is key! Moshe Feldenkrais has said something to the effect that we cannot change that of which we are not aware. So we'll begin with what may be most familiar, using imagery to support alignment.

IDEOKINESIS APPLIED TO PRINCIPLES OF MECHANICAL EFFICIENCY IN SKELETAL ALIGNMENT

Ideokinesis, a term coined by a piano teacher named Bonponsieve, combines "ideo," Greek for idea or thought, and movement, from "kinesis." Mabel Elsworth Todd, a modern pioneer in body-mind methods, was the first to use this term in reference to her work addressing postural and movement efficiency (Todd, 2018). It centered on using imagery as the mechanism for improving the way the body is organized in movement. Ideokinesis gives the mover a unified sense of form and energetic flow.

Standing alignment is instructed in a variety of ways. In this example, we'll use a felt sense of the body's anatomy, giving an image to guide an aligned natural standing posture.

When a structure's support is located near its center of gravity, less work or counterforce is needed to balance the structure's weight. The body's alignment follows this principle as well. The nearer the skeletal support is to the center of gravity the less muscular energy needs be exerted to maintain a position.

There are three main body weights to contend with in the standing position: the head, the chest or thorax, and the pelvis (Figure 3.1). For good alignment and its resulting efficient muscular use, these three weights should roughly stack one above the other. If thought of as blocks they could be shifted into a more mechanically advantageous place without changing any other features of their original position. Each of these blocks might also tilt side to side in the vertical dimension, roll forward to backward in the sagittal dimension, or rotate around its axis in the horizontal dimension, all leading to potential misalignment and therefore less efficient body use.

The body weights, thankfully, are not stacked blocks (however would we move?) but are connected and orchestrated by the spine. If we observe the spine in standing, we'll find five curves: the cranial, cervical, thoracic, lumbar, and sacrococcygeal. These curves flow forward and backward in the sagittal plane on a serpentine path. These five curves mediate the three main body weights of the head, thorax, and pelvis. When these curves are held "straight," tension results that reduces our spine's responsiveness and resilience. Most of the work we will do with clients' spines and torsos may be seen as addressing issues arising from the two lordotic (forward) curves of the cervical and lumbar spine. As the body's weight travels throughout the skeletal support structures, it's important to look locally as well as globally.

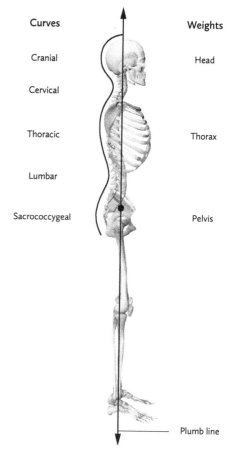

Figure 3.1 Skeleton of three body weights with plumb line

SOMATIC PRACTICE: Body weights and spinal curves

1. Lie on your back comfortably on the floor or a similar firm surface. Take a moment to release or yield your body's weight into gravity. Breathe diaphragmatically. Allow your body to rest.

2. When you are ready, bring your awareness to the parts of your body that are contacting the floor.

3. Now bring special attention to the back of your pelvis. Now the back of the ribs. And now the back of your head. Feel their weight and notice the differences between each of them, such as their size, volume, weightedness, etc.

4. When you are ready, bend your knees and bring the soles of your feet to the floor so your knees face upward comfortably. Press your heels into the floor to initiate a gentle rocking motion that moves up through your body to the top of your head. Release any holding in your body so that you can allow your three body weights to rock gently in a nodding motion. Notice the

rolling motion of your head, your chest, and your pelvis.

5. Next, push with one foot and then the other more slowly now, to tilt your pelvis with one hip higher than the other. Go side to side. Shift in your torso as well to produce this effect in your chest, and then lower one ear and then the other to tilt each body weight in the vertical dimension (using your body as the key to this orientation in space).

6. Now push with one foot and then the other to create a slight side-to-side rotating motion in your hips and pelvis. Do this as well by using your abdominals. Then gently and slowly turn your head side to side like in the gesture "no" but with your skull still weighted and against the floor. Notice the rotation in each of these three body weights.

7. Allow your legs to extend along the floor and notice how doing this changes the sagittal "roll" of the three body weights along the floor. Notice what this does to your cervical and lumbar spinal curves too. Bring the soles of the feet to the floor, bending the knees, and then extend the legs along the floor several times to explore these connections and differences.

8. When you are ready, roll to one side. Rest there, and then come to standing. Notice any changes in your body and awareness. Do you feel more or less ease?

A plumb line is a line used to find the vertical dimension in building or measuring depth. It usually has a small weight on the lower end so that true verticality can be perceived. While the spine isn't a straight line, the image and felt sense of a plumb line can be used as a way to orient the body in relation to the vertical dimension in the field of gravity to discern efficient standing alignment. The vertical midline alignment is our baseline orientation for all our movement and the orchestration of our limbs.

To contend with the challenge of efficient alignment of these three body weights and five spinal curves, we can use the bony landmarks in vertical standing as guides. They are:

- the side or back of ear
- the center of the side of the shoulder
- the center of the side of the rib cage
- the greater trochanter at the hip
- the center of the side of the knee
- the greater malleolus on the outside of the ankle.

SOMATIC PRACTICE: Vertical dimension plumb line for standing alignment

1. Begin by standing in a simple standing position. If the style of *yogasana* practice you do is natural, then stand in Mountain Pose, but if you add additional movements or tensions to this pose when doing it as instructed, simply stand. Relax your weight into gravity and notice your skeletal system providing you with the scaffolding to support your body's tissues in this upright position.

2. Bring awareness to the top of your head. If you like, use your hands to locate the uppermost "peak" of your skull while standing. Imagine and feel the plumb

line falling through the midline of your body.

3. Imagine this topmost part extending upward ever so slightly. If you like, actively reach this part upward while allowing the rest of your body to drape off it.

4. Now begin to make circles with the very top of your head leading upward. Allow the circles to become smaller and smaller so that you feel your body becoming even more centered and elongated. An image I use for this is a spiraled path circling a

mountain to its peak. Release this and circle again, in the opposite direction. Imagine a spiral line taking your peak. Now feel again your plumb line. Walk around and notice what you notice about your ease and efficiency of movement. Have you added anything extraneous like reaching forward with your chest? Are you still breathing diaphragmatically? This is something you can practice to increase your efficiency of use in standing alignment.

USING IDEOKINESIS FOR MECHANICAL EFFICIENCY

Supporting weight with efficient alignment is as necessary in practicing yoga *asana* and *vinyasa* as it is in performing the ordinary activities of daily life. The result of a force in any structure, whether it be the pull of gravity, acceleration, impact of an object, etc., is stress. The stress will be either compressional or it will be tensile. Compressive stress occurs when the external force compresses or pushes the components of the structure together. Tensile stress occurs when an external force pulls or stretches the structure's components apart. In simple standing our body's structure demonstrates both kinds of stress. In yoga practice gravity creates a wonderful variety of both types of stress throughout the body as it is oriented in and through the various planes of motion.

Mechanical balance is achieved when all forces acting on a structure are in balance. Stability increases as:

- the breadth of the base of support increases
- the axis of gravity passes closer to the center of gravity
- the center of weight is closer to the base, and
- the weight is distributed more evenly around the axis.

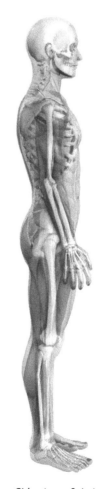

Figure 3.2 Side view of skeleton

When a structure is so stable that it can balance without outside support, it achieves mechanical balance. Our human body, with its intricately balanced weights, is not stable enough to achieve mechanical balance, nor would we want it to be! Neuromuscular activity and fascial tensile support give our skeletal structure the necessary tensegrity to maintain postural balance. Even though absolute mechanical balance is not possible for us, the more the center of our weight balances over our base of support the more efficient will be our use of energy in maintaining upright balance.

In the body you'll find three main supporting mechanical designs. Two are compressional and one is tensile. In the spinal column weight can sit in a stack. Even though, there are tensile elements to this anatomy. Another compressional design is a brace. We find the weight braced at the sacroiliac joints of the pelvis where the weight travels down the spine into the sacrum and the support of the legs arises from the ground into the ilia.

Additionally, the weight of the rib cage hangs off the front of the thoracic spine in a cantilever design. The weight of ribs is forward from the spine so it must be anchored by the spine and body. With these design elements at play, mechanical support can be improved by imaging and feeling elongation through the cervical and lumbar curves (Figure 3.2).

By having opposing curves, the spine is more flexible than a straight column and as such is more prone to collapse from the effects of gravity. The mechanical problem then is how to stabilize the spine without losing flexibility. Lengthening the spinal curves will establish support more closely to the axis of gravity. This reduces both stress on the spinal curves and the muscular effort needed to support the torso's weight.

SOMATIC PRACTICE: Spinal length for vertical mechanical efficiency

1. Stand in a natural standing position. You can also do this practice sitting.
2. Locate the place where your upper spine ends and your skull begins. Now imagine weight flowing down the spine from this place. Imagine this flow subtly elongating your spine, bringing space between your vertebrae and releasing your sacrum downward.
3. Picture the weight flowing all the way down to the ground. Let the sacrum hang downward into the space between the ilia. Allow the rest of your spine to follow. You can even see the sacrum as its five original vertebral segments, with space between them. Allow them to open downward. Picture a long dinosaur or kangaroo tail, heavy and substantial. You can also image downward-flowing warm water if you like, but include the sensation of weightedness.
4. Now from the base of your torso imagine energy, warm water, and lightness flowing upward along the front of your spine toward the same point where you began below your skull. Feel the upward lift and sense of suspension up the front of your spine.
5. Next, allow the base of your skull at the atlanto-occipital joint (AOJ) to open in the vertical dimension. Imagine a mouth there opening. Imagine energy flowing from there up the back of the head and over the top of it. Then let it flow downward over the face again to this juncture between the spine and skull.
6. At this place, allow the flow to continue again, down the back and up the front. The shape this will make is an elongated figure eight, with the lower loop longer than the upper one.

7. Keep this long figure eight in your mind as you take a walk, or stand if you've been sitting, or sit if you've been standing. What do you notice about your alignment?

Alignment and movement efficiency are intertwined. If the body is not aligned, muscular tension goes up, and movement efficiency is reduced. Better alignment gives us less muscle involvement for postural support, so more power is available for action. This in turn means greater capacity for work over a longer time.

CONSTRUCTIVE REST FOR SKELETAL ALIGNMENT

Mabel Elsworth Todd's Constructive Rest Position allows for body release and realignment in a supine position with legs bent and soles of the feet on the floor (Todd, 2008, pp. 289–290). The spine is passively elongated due to the pull of gravity, leaving the spinal discs to gently decompress. Similar to relaxation in *Shavasana*, this position allows for muscle tension reduction while the organs fall back toward the earth. The legs-bent position allows for greater decompression than in a typical *Shavasana*, although this can be a modification of the pose. Below is a version I once learned and have since been practicing nearly daily.

SOMATIC PRACTICE: Taking constructive rest

1. Lie on your back and bend your knees, placing the soles of the feet on the floor slightly wider than your knees. Turn the heels slightly outward and allow the knees to rest together at the midline, like you are making a pyramid. Be comfortable. Close your eyes.
2. Rest your arms on the floor or cross them on your chest.
3. Allow your weight to release into the field of gravity.
4. Allow the weight of your leg bones to travel downward from the knees, as if the knees were the top of a mountain and rivers were flowing down both sides toward your feet and toward your hips below.
5. As you remain comfortably in this position, your spine may elongate to the point that you will want to adjust your position to one of greater length along the floor. Go ahead and lift your head and reach it away from your body.
6. Five or ten minutes in this position is a good practice.

It's a good idea to roll onto your side before getting up. Once you stand and walk a bit, see what you notice.

GRAVITY AND SPACE IS OUR CONTEXT FOR LIVING

We begin our life's journey in an amniotic sea. As our bodies get bigger we relate to the uterine firmness all around our developing body structure. While in utero we experience the pull of gravity within the buoyancy of our ever-tightening oceanic container. Over the nine-month period we experience both the pressure of the womb, the pull of gravity, and then the powerful thrusting force of birth.

Without the external fluid support to which we've grown accustomed, we now struggle to gain control of our body in our new environment of gravity and space. We must learn to contend with the constant pull of gravity on our bodily form in three-dimensional space.

Throughout our first year we seem propelled, milestone by milestone, toward uprightness. We orient in space according to the pull of gravity and learn fundamentally which way is up and which is down. This primary sense of the vertical dimension gives us an awareness of our midline. This is the central axis around which we will orient and continue to coordinate our movements.

We discover new ways to move away from and back into the pull of the earth. Mother Earth herself teaches us how to differentiate our bodily selves and then merge again with her powerful attractive force. As we gain skill in mediating between these, exerting away from and returning into gravity, we gain strength, coordination, balance, and agility.

The manner in which we mobilize our body's weight to traverse space and terrain in order to satisfy our needs and curiosity creates a template upon which we continue to organize our future learning experiences. Yoga *asana* and *vinyasa* practice is an extraordinary way to visit and revisit the history of our embodied learning experiences.

Hatha is a combination of two words, *ha*, meaning sun, and *tha*, meaning moon. This does not only refer to the external sun and moon in the heavens but to these inner attitudes within us. The *ha* or sun principle is experienced through activation, assertion, and willfulness, while the *tha* or moon principle is characterized by receptive, passive, and accepting experiences. *Ha* is often equated with the masculine force in nature and *tha* with the feminine. Hatha yoga expresses the union of two fundamental aspects of nature, similar to the Tao expressing the relationship between yin and yang.

SOMATIC PRACTICE: Coping with the environment of gravity and space

1. Lie on your back. Release your weight to rest on the earth without effort. Find comfort.
2. Notice what parts of your body rest on the floor. Notice which parts hang back to the floor. Notice where you feel the architecture of your bony supports: the skull, the rib cage, the pelvis, the shapes of the arms and hands, the shapes of the legs and feet. Feel their volume.
3. Feel how the breath may shape your body's position, ever so slightly, and, in doing so, change where the weight falls.
4. Allow your arms to float upward toward the ceiling. Notice what happens to your weight distribution as you do so. Does it shift even slightly? Let the arm lift turn into a reach. Reach into the space around your body. (The space that you can reach to in a stationary position is called "reach space.") Rest.
5. Allow your legs to float upward toward

the ceiling. Notice what happens to your weight as you do so. Does it shift slightly or a lot? Let this turn into a reach. Reach into the space around your body with one or both of your legs. Explore the space into which you can reach.

6. Place your hands and feet on the floor. Push into the floor. Push and see if you can lift any part of your torso off the floor. How about your head? Roll to a different surface, place a different side of your body in contact with the floor. Push again. Explore.

7. See what, if any, other parts you can use to push and lift off the floor. Try a few different ways.

8. Now take your time and experiment with lifting one of the three main body weights (of head, chest, pelvis), your head. Notice what you do to lift it. How does your weight change? Do you hold somewhere else? What do you feel as you lift? Do you notice any changes in the relationship of your jaw to your skull? What does this remind you of? Rest.

9. Now experiment with lifting your chest. Notice what you do to lift it. Does your weight change? Do you hold somewhere else? What do you feel as you lift? Does this remind you of anything familiar? Do you like this? Is it hard or easy? Rest.

10. Now take your time and experiment with lifting your pelvis. Notice what you need to do to lift it. Does your weight change?

Do you hold somewhere else? What do you feel as you lift? Does this remind you of anything? Do you like this? Is it hard or easy? Rest.

11. Roll to another surface. Release your weight so you are resting on the earth without effort. Make yourself comfortable.

12. Notice what parts of your body rest on the floor. Notice which parts hang back to the floor. Notice where you feel the architecture of your bony supports: the skull, the rib cage, the pelvis, the shapes of the arms and hands, the shapes of the legs and feet.

13. Feel how the breath shapes your body's position, changing perhaps where the weight falls.

14. Now repeat the exploration of lifting head, then chest, then pelvis as you did above.

15. Roll to a different surface of your body. Explore yielding into the floor so you can activate and push and reach and lift other body parts up off the floor. If you would like to travel in space, i.e., move somewhere else with these actions, do so.

16. Notice what parts of your body rest on the floor. Notice which parts hang back to the floor. Now roll to another surface that you have not used as a support. Repeat yielding, and pushing and reaching and lifting, and notice if you like traveling or not. Notice what you notice. Take your time. And when you are ready, rest. Take a moment to allow your nervous system to record the experience your cells have had.

DYNAMIC ALIGNMENT THROUGH SOMATIC PRINCIPLES

Dynamic alignment refers to ongoing neuromuscular adjustment of body areas in movement for the purpose of high-level function. Visualization and guidance as to what to sense while visualizing is a workable means to repatterning for optimal body use.

Awareness is key as is having a good enough map of the territory of the body as its moves and supports the transfer of weight through space. My experience is that when imagery is tied to sound biomechanical concepts, with a clear enough embodied understanding of the anatomy in question, not only can the presenting issue be dealt with, but the client's range of movement, strength, and body organization will be improved, as will their somatic awareness.

JOINT CENTRATION

Joint centration is the maintenance of favorable alignment of a joint through its range of motion. This requires the optimal mechanical position of a joint through its range, preventing wear and tear on the articulating surfaces of the bones involved.

Pain, injury, and impairment often result from inadequate mechanical support for the lines of force traveling through the body in movement. While standing alignment may look good, in motion, patterns of global body use as well as movement phrasing will impact the area or joint in question.

Although clients may expect a quick fix or exercises targeted on the problem area, say the ankle, this joint may be stressed due to an imbalance of forces converging there due to weakness, tightness, and faulty movement patterning elsewhere in the body. Yoga therapists often need to educate their clients as to the longer-term arc of work to address the various elements present in an injury or chronic musculoskeletal condition. Finding ways to embody mechanical principles in motion can provide the balanced coordination needed to pattern alignment throughout a wide range of movement possibilities.

COMPLEMENTARY MOVEMENT OF BONES MAKING UP A JOINT

The mechanical principle explored here is focused on the knee joint but can be applied to any joint. Complementary movement of the two (or more) bones that make up a joint is a Body-Mind Centering® concept that is well worth embodying. For this practice, we'll work with two parts of this concept somatically (Cohen, 2012, pp. 18–25).

The first part has to do with the joint surfaces meeting in the joint and the observation that most joint surfaces will present as either concave or convex, irrespective of their joint classification. One bone of the pair will be more ball-like while the other will be more socket-like.

Like a spaceship orbiting the earth, the socket-like bone in the joint will travel (excursion) around the ball-like bone in the joint. And, like the earth, the ball-like bone will also rotate, and this will be in an opposite direction. Countersupport arises from the equality of force this provides. The counterbalancing of forces of both moving bones allows the joint space to remain even through the joint's range of motion. The axis of the movement will be in the center of the convex ball surface.

The second part has to do with perceiving the bones as levers. This involves sensing both ends of the bone in question and feeling the force translate through the bone from one end to another in joint action. For instance, say I am working with my knee, and I wish to strengthen its use and find more support. If I stand from sitting in a chair and only sense my femur and tibia at my knee, I have a more hinge-like localized experience and the movement does not feel very stable, well-coordinated, or strong.

To bring more skeletal support with greater centration, I find both ends of my femur, the distal and proximal, and both ends of my tibia (I recognize the fibula is also at play but for this explanation, I'm leaving it out). Then, as I go to stand, weight-shifting from the seat over my feet, I lever them thus:

- I feel the proximal end of my femurs move forward as the distal ends move back, and
- I feel the distal ends of my tibias move forward as their proximal ends move back. Try it! What do you notice?

An ideokinetic image from the work of Body-Mind Centering® fortunately brings to some degree these two awareness strategies together. In it we envision two cogwheels at the articulating ends of the two moving bones in the joint. A cogwheel is a wheel or sphere that rolls in the opposite direction to its neighbor. Think of gears rolling at the joint, functioning to keep space even between the bones as they move.

SOMATIC PRACTICE: Joint centration

1. We'll explore the cogwheel image in the lower extremity. It works equally well with the upper extremity, which you are invited to explore using this same somatization.
2. Begin resting supine. Feel your legs and focus on your hip, knee, and ankle joints.
3. Imagine a gear at each hip joint, made up of two cogwheels with their teeth or cogs interfacing. Flex and extend slightly at each hip and feel the countermotion of the ilium and femur. This naturally happens. To focus on and support this action with imagery will help with joint centration.
4. Next, imagine a gear at each knee joint, made up of two cogwheels, their teeth or cogs interfacing. Flex and extend slightly at each knee and feel the countermotion of the femur and tibia. This naturally happens. To focus on and support this action with imagery will help with joint centration.

5. Now imagine a gear at each ankle joint, made up of two cogwheels, their teeth or cogs interfacing. Flex and extend slightly at each ankle and feel the countermotion of the tibia–fibula and the talus bone. This naturally happens. To focus on and support this action with imagery will help with joint centration.
6. Now feel both legs with these cogwheels active. Move as you would like while working to orchestrate the counter rotations in the leg joints. Find a way to stand, keeping this awareness and ideokinetic image going. Walk, dance, jog, and otherwise move about your space, paying attention to the feedback from your joints. What do you feel in terms of support? Is the spatial clarity and sense of dimensionality helpful? How do your knees feel?

THE BODY'S VARIOUS DIAPHRAGMS IN RELATION TO THE *LINGAS*

There are numerous views concerning the body's diaphragms. For our purposes, we'll consider a diaphragm to be an organization of somewhat flexible tissue into a potential dome-shaped structure in the physical body. Among other functions, a diaphragm gives dynamic support to nearby perpendicular physical structures. It may also provide a resonant tympanic structure for sound and energy.

Alignment through the body's diaphragms is relational. We can find a fluidly mobile stacking of the horizontally oriented ones in standing, or we may consider how they each relate one to another without reference to gravity.

The body's diaphragms from lower to upper are:

- soles of the feet
- palms of the hands (in quadruped position)
- abdominal wall (in quadruped position)
- pelvic floor
- breathing (thoracic) diaphragm
- thoracic inlet

- larynx and vocal folds
- hard and soft palate at roof of mouth
- cranial vault (calvaria).

In my exploration of the body's diaphragms I've found it useful to divide them into three groups: (1) those pertaining to the upper, namely the thoracic inlet, the voice, the palate, and the cranium; (2) those pertaining to the hands and feet; and (3) those pertaining to the torso, namely the breathing diaphragm, the abdominal wall, and the pelvic floor.

If a diaphragm functions not only as a structural support but also as a permeable barrier we might ask what it impedes. In the yoga tradition there may not be a physical substance limited by these enclosures; however, at the energetic level there is symbolic language that represents some containment for the areas between them.

THE *LINGAS* AND *GRANTHIS*

The three symbolic *lingas* in the body act as subtle barriers to progressively higher levels of unitive consciousness in my experience. At the pelvic floor diaphragm and Muladhara Chakra is the Svayambu Linga. It is sometimes related to Brahma Granthi. The *granthis* are known to be physical-metaphysical "knots" or limitations of consciousness and energy. What I share here is my experience of them as containers of energetic seas that have an emotional tone or coloring and a set of psychophysical concerns.

At this level in the body, Brahma Granthi holds the life energy in the body and is related to concerns of survival, safety, and having enough to live. The energetic sea it preserves rises above this area and is contained from above by the next superior barrier at the thoracic diaphragm. The energy contained in this region functions to preserve individual life in the material sense. It is associated with the waking state (*jagrat*), and

the syllable "A" in the universal mantra of Om (AUM). Of many other options, a familiar yoga practice called *Mula bandha* (root lock) to some degree works to facilitate progress with Brahma Granthi.

Svayambu Linga, however, is within the Shushumna Nadi and as such is the domain of Shakti herself. A practitioner of yoga can do what they can to create the proper conditions for advancement, but it is up to the Divine within as to whether advancement will take place.

At the heart center, at Anahata Chakra, is Bana Linga. It is related to Vishnu Granthi, the second knot between the Anahata Chakra at the heart and the Ajna Chakra, at the third eye slightly above and between the eyebrows according to my experience. The energetic sea in this area is colored by concerns for enacting what it is we think about and desire. It can take us into an internal state of imagination, dreams, ideals, and strategies. It is associated with the dream state (*svapna*), and the syllable "U" in the universal mantra of Om (AUM). Among many other practices, the commonly known practice of *Uddiyana bandha* (abdominal lock) works to facilitate progress here.

Itara Linga, at the third eye or Ajna Chakra, relates to Rudra Granthi. The energetic sea here is bounded by Ajna Chakra below the highest central point or *bindu* of the Saharara Chakra just above the top of the head. My experience of this region is that it is colored by the glimpse of the transcendent and draws us ever closer to yoga's goal and all that comes with leaving behind what we know in that transition. This energy sea is associated with the deep sleep state (*sushupti*) and the syllable "M" in the universal mantra of Om (AUM). Among many other practices, the commonly known practice of *Jaladhara bandha* (chin lock) works to facilitate progress here.

SOMATIC PRACTICE: Dynamic alignment through the body's diaphragms

1. Begin standing and notice your sense of verticality and support in the vertical dimension. Notice the leveling of all the horizontal diaphragms: the soles of the feet, the pelvic floor, the thoracic diaphragm, the thoracic inlet, the larynx, the palates, and the cranial vault.

2. With awareness of the top cranium and palate, begin to roll down your spine by nodding yes and then allowing the downward movement of the head to lead you to slowly release your chin to your throat. Feel the change in the larynx.

3. As if you are releasing one vertebra at a time into gravity, continue to slowly soften forward. Feel the thoracic inlet tumble forward. The arms will hang.

4. At the point where you will next release the thoracic or breathing diaphragm forward, begin to allow the knees to bend slightly so your low back rounds instead of hinging from the hips to fold from there. As well, allow your sacrum to be heavy.

5. Pause with the pelvic floor diaphragm still in its initial horizontal plane relationship with gravity and allow the weight of the upper to balance against the weight of the pelvis and grounding of the legs before continuing. Relax whatever you can here.

6. Then release this position and allow the tail and sit bones to rise behind you so that the pelvic floor diaphragm might also tilt forward. Notice what you notice. Remain here as long as you like.

7. Then bend your knees and begin the roll up slowly, allowing and noticing each diaphragm as it comes into its horizontal plane relationship with gravity.

8. Keep the chin down on the front of the throat as you align the larynx. Then feel the palate and the cranium return to the horizontal plane to complete the practice.

What do you notice?

EXPLORING TONE IN THE BODY'S DIAPHRAGMS

A diaphragm is a thin, somewhat taut, flexible partition. It can consist of a single material or of various parts that act as a divider. The body's various diaphragms do not consist of the same tissues in their composition. While they are all not the same structurally, they do share some defining features. One is that the overall tone or level of activation in the body affects their tautness depending, of course, on several factors. There are several ways to look at tone, but generally it is the level of activation of any system when not being called upon. It is like an idling position of an engine—on but not in gear. Muscle tone may be the most familiar version of tone. We've learned it is the continuous passive partial contraction of muscle tissue in its resting state.

Our nervous system has in place many automatic patterns of responsiveness that help us regulate and modulate our reactions. These patterns of response can be tuned to our internal perceptual environment, and to our external environment including the objects and the people in it. We're auto tuned, you might say, to kinds of touch, to sound, volume, and timbre, and to proximity in space. We're also programmed to respond to changes in our position in relation to gravity.

Our autonomic tone has to do with the balance of activation of the sympathetic and parasympathetic divisions of the autonomic nervous system. Its job is primarily to keep us in the game of life! It maintains homeostasis and balance overall. It also activates specific aspects of our being to respond to signals of threat or safety in our experience beneath our conscious awareness. While not the focus of this work, Stephen Porges' polyvagal theory has provided a sophisticated way to organize and discuss autonomic awareness and perception of states before and beyond words that relate to our level of inner and outer engagement.

The autonomic system can produce higher and lower tone states with regard to maintaining a state of alert readiness, social engagement, feigning-death shutdown, or a release of that state into maintenance and rest. Nuanced strategies for survival can then arise from these autonomic pathways. The autonomic system's active–passive polarity reflects an earlier one noted: that of pushing away from and returning to gravity in our first year so as to organize ourselves in movement. We do a dance of going out into our world and returning inward to ourselves throughout our day, week, and lifetime. For this our body adjusts so as to ready us to meet our world. Then we can release our outward focus, allowing for return to our own inner world. We may have a higher overall base tone, or a lower overall base tone, something like a "vibe" that is our own way of being in the world.

We may also have an injury or an illness affecting an organ or specific area of the body that affects its ability to function. It will then have a different tone than the rest of the body. The various diaphragms likewise may have differing levels of tone depending on several factors. Our overall tone, illness, or injury, the contents of the *granthis* they manage, the habitual or sustained use of that part of the body, and the overall liveliness of the body systems involved will each have a role.

Working with yoga postures and *vinyasa* movements can modulate the tone of the diaphragms, taking them into higher or lower levels of activation. Exercising this dynamism of activation helps us find support without rigidity and ease without collapse.

I invite you to use propped restorative practices in various orientations to gravity to explore how you might reduce the tone (stretch, elongate, and release) of tissues involved in any diaphragm in question. Explore finding ways to activate the tissues through vibration, sound, rebounding, quick weight shifts, changes of direction, and through pressure. Perhaps one of the most valuable things about yoga *asana* and *vinyasa* practice is that the movements of pose-counterpose, bending the body one way and then the opposite way, go far in the way of modulating the tone of the tissues involved.

Please also investigate doing some postures and *vinyasa* movements while paying attention to the tone of the diaphragms involved. For instance, study the resilience and activity of your breathing diaphragm before and after doing a series of standing side bends going to one side and back to vertical, then the other side and back to vertical, with breath coordination, several times. This is just one possibility. There are many more. How do the body's diaphragms reflect your ability to move with ease from inner and outer environs? How do they play a part in your ability to modulate your capacity to meet the demands of life with authenticity and present-moment responsiveness?

LANGHANA AND *BRAHMANA* AS A SOMATIC BASIS FOR TRAVELING INWARD AND OUTWARD

A rhythm develops in the early weeks of life in utero that organizes various body parts into a whole-body experience. This rhythm is based on two primary patterns in our human make-up that are manifest throughout the pulse of the entire universe. The vocabulary of Ayurveda and yoga uses the terms *langhana* and *brahmana*. They refer to the properties of condensing and expanding respectively, and are used in various contexts.

An inherent dynamic exists between these two patterns, as in all of nature. Our autonomic nervous system holds the subtle baseline of this alternating rhythm. There is always a rhythm of expansion and condensing going on in the body in general, and very specifically in many of the body's functions such as in breathing, the heartbeat, and the flow of cerebrospinal fluid; together condensing and expanding form a baseline rhythm of interchange that can be seen as a subtext for all later movements and interaction patterns. This rhythm can be experienced as one of moving out from self or expanding, and one of returning in or condensing. I call this "The Big In and the Big Out." It includes all that happens and can be experienced along the way.

This rhythm can be experienced on a continuum of polarities of expanding and condensing, asserting and withdrawing, opening and closing, moving toward or away, gathering and scattering, being up and ready to go or being tired and ready to rest. All manner of polar rhythmic gradated change can be reflected upon them in this exchange.

Our ability to skillfully engage with our world requires a rhythmic exchange so that we can continue to function optimally. Health issues, learning issues, emotional imbalance, and general exhaustion of the adult population can be connected to this need for a rhythmic exchange from internal to external states of being. Even though this is a whole-self experience, it may be that parts of oneself may not participate in the exchange. For instance, an injured body area may not be comfortable expanding along with other areas. Or one may experience being outward in some parts of oneself while inward in other parts. Another possibility is being stuck somewhere on the continuum, unable to move inward or outward in either direction.

We can learn to attend to, feel, and be present to what is happening and how our body and its autonomic system sets us up for responding. Or we can ignore, cover up with other patterns, and not take the time to allow such deeper processes to come into awareness. Exploring the continuum of "The Big In and the Big Out" gives opportunity to gain experiential insight into how we pattern ourselves to meet and interact with the world around us. Are we ready? Do we have the support we require? Are we able to move to where we need to be? Can we meet the world with openness and responsiveness? What is not effective in how we engage? Are we organized enough to be efficient in our exchanges? Are there impediments or inhibitions in our patterns of relating?

Yoga practice can be a way to open to ourselves at these subtle, yet physical ways of relating to our environment. This is at the heart of somatic work, of which yoga is one systematic approach. Our individual manner of moving inward and outward relies on this foundational rhythm.

SOMATIC PRACTICE: Yoga's *langhana* and *brahmana*

This practice evolved out of "The Big In and the Big Out" somatic practice in Chapter 2, where it was used to experience, to some degree, the way our autonomic nervous system organizes us to attend inwardly and outwardly. When we think of alignment, it's usually in relation to body position in the field of gravity, and whether supporting structures are well enough aligned. We in essence bond to the earth and then use this as a basis for moving away from it with its support. Prior to that, in utero we have the potential to bond to self, i.e., to be at home and comfortable while inwardly focused. We may have had difficulty in utero, at birth, and at other times during our lives and this has interfered with our ability to find comfort in our own self-referencing awareness. Alternatively, we may have found that this interior experiential world is the only place we feel safe and at home. Or we may have had any number of experiences between these two extremes. These experiences can be felt in our body as we move from one extreme to the other and will affect our movement and expressive range, and possible vocabulary of effective action. As well, our ability to support ourselves in our engagement with the world with vitality and presence may be seen in this continuum.

We may wish to further explore our patterns of interaction as we traverse the dynamism between self, world, and those in it, after doing this initial exploration. Moving from retreating and condensing inward, or medial rotation, flexion, and adduction, to advancing and expanding outward, or lateral rotation, extension, and abduction allows us to traverse the spatial ranges that organize our gradated movement in three-dimensional space. This allows us to locate the primary neuromuscular connections needed to support the actions of modulating our tone through near and far reach-space in movement.

1. Begin standing. You may also wish to try this sitting as you may get different information. Notice your posture, particularly where you are supported and well integrated and ready for movement in any direction at any moment. How connected to your center do you feel? Do you feel "hooked-up" from center to periphery, and able to move from where you are with ease? Please notice what you notice of this starting position.

2. Move your body toward its center, condensing and rounding inward in any way that suits you. Go as far as you can in this direction. It's okay if this takes you to the floor, or if you bend your knees fully or the like. Bring your senses in, pull your energy inward, attend inwardly and let the outside go. Notice if this reminds you of anything: retreating, protecting yourself, taking cover, curling up after a long day. Do you generally feel ease in doing this? Are there any parts of you, i.e., your body, your senses and awareness not coming along? What comes up for you?

3. Now move outward returning to what you remember your starting position to be. What changes in your body's level of connection do you notice? What else do you notice?

4. Now move outward away from your body's center, expanding, extending, and reaching out in any way that suits you. Go as far as you

can in this direction. Move into a big, wide position within your capacity. What is this like? Notice if this reminds you of anything: expanding, revealing yourself, greeting others, being seen, taking space. Do you generally feel ease in doing this? Do you feel strong and agile in this position or disconnected and overextended, or something else? Are there any parts of you, i.e., your body, your senses and awareness not coming along? Are they places of disintegration, like abdominals or core support or shoulder movement inhibition? What comes up for you?

5. Now move inward and return to your starting position. What changes in your body's level of connection do you notice? What else do you notice?

6. Repeat moving in and out as you like. Try this from a seated position as well if you'd like to investigate any difference from the seated position.

7. Rest when you are done exploring. Take time to transition out of the somatization. Perhaps jot down any notes for further reflection and sharing.

Understanding one's own relationship with condensing and expanding movement in space gives insight into autonomic tone. The body's diaphragms reflect our overall tone and our current embodiment of tone in specific areas. Tone responds to internal and external environmental factors. The practice of yoga *asana* and *vinyasa* movement expands our capabilities in responsiveness and ease by modulating tone. This can lead to greater resilience and freedom of expression during life's continuous barrage of encounters.

USING ECCENTRIC ACTION FOR DYNAMIC ALIGNMENT

Returning to the notion of alignment, we must consider the position of body parts in space in relation to gravity. What mechanical stresses are being put on the body's tissues? Is this particular position of hopeful balance of efficient use? Where movement is concerned, dynamic alignment comes into play in which forces are directed throughout the body as it moves, still in the field of gravity but at times in defiance of it.

We again consider use and efficiency but in motion there is so much more at play. Often the reminders we use for standing alignment, i.e., the imagery or directions we've learned, come to naught as our movement needs for quick weight shifts and directional changes, such as in playing tennis or soccer, or even walking a leashed dog that suddenly lurches, takes us out of the potted plant imagery of static alignment.

Some features of movement can come in handy here, such as focusing on one side of the bone in movement, say on the eccentric lengthening contraction versus the concentric one. Imaging length and sensing for support can help one guide in lowering into gravity quite well. It can also give a sense of lightness to movement as well as length and space to the joint when used as a somatic directive. Dancers are often taught to lift from underneath when brushing the leg out and up in a *grand battement*, for example.

SOMATIC PRACTICE: Limb lift

1. Stand. If you have a full-length mirror, please face it.

2. Feel the top of your thigh where your quadriceps are located. Imagine them contracting along with your hip flexors to lift your entire leg with the knee extended forward as high as you comfortably can, keeping the rest of your body neutral. Allow the leg to slowly lower, feeling the work of the quads as it comes down.

3. Now imagine the back of the leg from your hip to the heel as a long stretchy line. Imagine this line lengthening outward away from your hip in space, stretching along the arc-like pathway as you now lift the leg again. Then let it come down.

What was the difference in your experience? Was one tighter in your hip? Was one more spacious and freeing? Was one easier than the other?

Another possibility for alignment that is not musculoskeletally based but that influences these tissues greatly is the felt sense of the organs. Most of the time our internal organs function beneath our awareness; it's usually only when there's a problem with one of them that we may become more acutely aware of their location. Our overall wellness requires our organ system to be vital as it carries out the functions necessary to our internal survival. In the torso primarily this involves breathing, acceptance of nourishment, and elimination. Experienced yogis who practice *asana* and *vinyasa* develop an intimacy with all the parts of their bodies, and this is also true of the organs. Certain *asana* and *vinyasa* practices manipulate the organs and use them at times for weight-bearing compressional or suspended tensile support due to the various levels, planes, and body areas engaged over the course of a practice session.

A way of considering their role in alignment from Body-Mind Centering© is that the organs are the "contents" within the skeletal-flesh "container" (Cohen, 2012, pp. 28–53). An image that came to me is that of a jelly donut or any pastry with a crème filling. When you pick up a fresh jelly donut, it is pliable and flexible, and you can feel the filling inside. You have a sense its voluminous innards are softer than the dough. Without the filling, the dough would collapse inward and flatten a bit in your hand. In this same way, the "jelly-like" organs provide volume and substance to the donut of your musculoskeletal system. Of course, this is a simplified impression. We know that there are structures within organs and that they have membranes and exhibit higher or lower tone. Yet their tonus and form can provide a sense of bulk, dimension, and presence experientially, which then supports the body's movement through space functionally.

Just as our skeletal-muscular system guides our external movement through space, organs occupy our inner space and therefore can be experienced as guiding our internal movement. The organs express our inner motivations; our skeletal-muscular system provides the structure for their outward expression. And while our bones align and move us through the environment, our organs provide the internal integrity for that alignment. Muscles provide the visible forces for the mobility of our bones; organs can be experienced as providing the internal patterning that contributes to the organization and patterning of muscular coordination.

Attending consciously to one's organs and moving from there may be unfamiliar to most people. But yogis are familiar with this feeling as the practice of *asana* and *vinyasa* relies heavily on the manipulation and support of the organs during the weight-bearing support for positions and actions taking place in the various planes of movement. Inviting individuals to explore work at this deep internal physiological level may open them up to physical and mental horizons and resources heretofore left behind. As Linda Hartley writes in *Wisdom of the Body Moving*,

"contacting and moving from the organs can give support, energy, power, feeling and presence to posture, movement, and vocal expression. Holding patterns in the body and mind can be gently released, allowing fluidity and expansiveness to return to our movement" (1995, p. 204).

Attending consciously to one's organs and initiating moving from the space they occupy may be unfamiliar to most people. This exploration may feel strange at first, but because we have seen deep holding patterns release with awareness and embodiment of these tissues, please suspend the rational functioning of your questioning mind as you can and give this somatization a try.

SOMATIC PRACTICE: Organ exploration

1. Begin by looking at some anatomy images of the organ system and organs, and note their general locations. See where your interest lies. Then...
2. Lie on the floor in a comfortable position and breathe easily.
3. Simply notice your breathing without judgment or conscious interference.
4. Allow the weight of your bones to fall into gravity.
5. What do you notice by consciously releasing your bones into the earth?
6. Has this releasing of bones affected your breathing?
7. Allow the weight of your organs to fall into gravity. As you release your organs into the earth, how is your breathing affected?
8. Now bring attention to your skull and sense and imagine the location of your brain within it. See if you can get a sense of the brain as an organ. What is its size, where are its boundaries? Feel its density, its energy. Notice what you notice. Now see if you can initiate movement from the brain. Rotate around the vertical axis. Move side to side in the vertical plane. Nod up and down from the brain around a horizontal axis. Move, feel, and rest as you like.
9. Move to your sinuses and mouth. Now see if you can follow first your trachea down through your vocal diaphragm and into your lungs. Feel the top lobe, the middle, the lower lobe of the right lung. Now feel the top and lower lobe of the left lung. Sense your heart. See if you can move from the location of the heart. Rotate it to the left. Now to the right. Can you rotate the heart left with the lungs going to the right? Tilt, nod, and play with moving the heart. Move, feel, and rest as you like.
10. Now let's move into the stomach, below the diaphragm and a bit to the left side. Follow it into the small intestine in the pelvis. See if you can find the sense of it. And now the large intestine, coming up the right, across a bit below the waist, down the left, and snaking out to the anus. Move, feel, and rest as you like.
11. When you are ready, slowly find a comfortable way to gently roll to your side, to balance on one side with knees bent like you might sleep. Make yourself comfortable.

12. See what it is like to initiate some small movement from your digestive system. Do some gentle movement. Now find a way to rock gently back and forth. Do this for a minute or longer. Just give it a go. Eyes closed is good. Move, feel, and rest as you like.

13. Now find an organ that interests you, like the liver, spleen, pancreas, or maybe the kidneys or bladder. See if you can locate within your body the size and boundaries of that organ. Where is it clear? Where is it not so clear? See if you can initiate movement. Rotate, tilt, nod, or find other movement that occurs organically. See if this movement will translate into a larger movement in more than this one area of your body.

14. Now let that go, pause a moment. Now roll to a different surface, either back or front.

15. Where in your body did you initiate your movement transition? How did the movement progress through your body?

16. How did your external movement through space reflect that path of movement through your internal space?

17. What organs lie along this pathway?

18. Breathe easily. Rest.

19. Now focus on some organ, or the entire organ system within the body. When you are ready, repeat each sound on a long exhale with me: first A, then U, then M. Here we go, ahhhhh. Now, oooooooo. Now, mmmmmm. What resonance in the organs do you notice? One more time... A–U–M.

20. When you are ready, notice how you feel. What differences do you notice?

21. Return to the group or remain where you are.

SOMATIC PRACTICE: Ratioed breathing from the organs

This exploration is a bit more complex. I feel it bridges the physical sheath with the energetic one, but that is my perception. You may find a different way of describing it. Bonnie Bainbridge Cohen taught that the muscles follow the bones, and the bones will follow the organs. I worked to understand this in my own body. My experience included an awareness of the energetic sheath as a sort of power grid that kept the frequencies of the various body tissues humming within their own harmonic ranges. When the breath was applied to the organ energy, using the principles of *langhana* and *brahmana*, usefulness relating to postural integrity came into view.

We'll begin with a lung exploration as it is directly affected by breath, quickly changed, and relatively easy to feel. If you would like, pull up an image of the lungs and look at them before beginning this exploration. This practice can be done with other organs and with non-symmetrical pairs of them.

Part 1 Creating asymmetry

1. Breathe evenly, noticing the action of air moving in both lungs.

2. Now focus attention on the left lung only and inhale for approximately twice as long as you exhale. If this is not comfortable, simply make the inhale a tad longer by slightly shortening the exhale and increasing the length of the inhale a bit.

3. Imagine/feel the breath initiation from the left lung itself. As you inhale, feel the lung's expansion into space; as you exhale just exhale. Continue for five breaths. You can do more than this, but we'll keep it to five for this exploration.

4. Now bring your awareness to the right lung; feel yourself breathing in this lung.

5. Now exhale twice as long as you inhale. If this is not comfortable, simply make the exhale a tad longer by slightly shortening the inhale and increasing the length of the exhale a bit.

6. As you do so, focus on condensing this lung as you exhale. When you inhale for half as long do nothing in terms of size. Repeat for a total of five breaths.

7. Notice the shape of your upper torso or thorax area. Notice the alignment of your spine. Do you notice any aspect of it being off-midline or center?

Part 2 Coming back to symmetry

1. Beginning where you left off in Part 1, focus again on the right lung and inhale for approximately twice as long as you exhale. If this is not comfortable, simply make the inhale a tad longer by slightly shortening the exhale and increasing the length of the inhale a bit.

2. Imagine/feel the breath initiation from the right lung itself. As you inhale, feel the lung's expansion into space; as you exhale, just exhale. Continue for five breaths.

3. Now bring your awareness to the left lung; feel yourself breathing in this lung.

4. Now exhale twice as long as you inhale. If this is not comfortable, simply make the exhale a tad longer by slightly shortening the inhale and increasing the length of the exhale a bit.

5. As you do so, focus on condensing this lung as you exhale. When you inhale for half as long do nothing in terms of size. Repeat for a total of five breaths.

6. Notice the shape of your upper torso or thorax area. Notice the alignment of your spine. Do you notice a balance of size and volume through the lungs? Has the spine in this area returned to midline or center? If not, explore what is needed for this to happen.

7. Repeat with the opposite side, expanding and condensing respectively.

CHAPTER 4

Embodying Use of Space

The last chapter's focus was on static and dynamic alignment. In this chapter we look at an embodied understanding of space as one aspect of stopping down the process of observation of self or other when questioning alignment and well-organized bodily use for movement efficiency.

THE VALUE OF THREE-DIMENSIONAL SPACE

What we're seeing and sensing when we assess efficient use are body parts: bone, muscle, ligament, etc., organized in space. From this we determine whether their posture and organization are functional, or if they are wanting in some way. Then we figure out how and what to do about that, and how we are going to do it. From this understanding we go forward into the best ways to teach that particular person in that particular case. Leaving that off for now and returning to the first issue of correct observation, having a clear view of what is where in space is the first step.

In Chapter 1 we discussed Rudolph Laban's space notation for orienting and tracking movement in space. Here we'll apply that understanding to the practice of Functional Movement Rehabilitation™ in yoga therapy. Within this work we draw upon three interrelated categories I call the Three Categories of Correctives. They are:

- *Differentiation*: Having to do with range of motion, mobility in the right places, flexibility, and articulation of movement capacity.

- *Support*: Having to do with tissue integrity and muscular strength, enough stability in the right places, and control through the effective range of motion.
- *Organization*: Having to do with how the body is coordinated and orchestrated in action and movement phrasing and sequences. In Functional Movement Rehabilitation™'s Three Streams, concerning organization we focused on:
  - *local action patterning*: having to do with efficiency of neuromuscular action of a localized body part or area.
  - *global action patterning*: having to do with efficiency of neuromuscular action regarding the whole body.
  - *integrative movement skill patterning*: having to do with refinement of total body use and local action with respect to an efficient and effective enactment of a specific movement task, goal, or set of goals.

To illustrate the value of astute spatial awareness beyond the theoretical and into practicality, I'll share a somatization for each of the Three Categories of Correctives listed above.

SPATIAL CLARITY IN ACTION

Differentiation

Differentiation is an important factor in movement rehabilitation in that for efficient movement to take place each body part should be able to move in its optimal pathway in space or hold in its optimal position. The body parts need to have the freedom to do so and must be coordinated correctly, which leads to organization (see below). Dissociation generally means the disconnection or separation of something from something else. Regarding the body, it has to do with the bones in a joint each having the ability to move independently. How do we tell this? We see their movement in *space*.

Irmgard Bartenieff, a physical therapist, dancer, and pioneer of dance therapy, was a student of Laban. She applied her training to rehabilitation during the polio epidemic and beyond, codifying a series of movements called the Basic Six, within her larger method of Bartenieff Fundamentals, that encapsulated a host of spatial and dynamic movement, and kinesiological concepts.

SOMATIC PRACTICE: Thigh lift from Bartenieff's Basic Six

In this movement the goal is to flex the hip and lift the bent leg off the floor in the most efficient way possible. Are they able to do this simple action with minimal effort, little extraneous or compensatory movement or "bracing," and with activation primarily of the iliopsoas without superficial muscular involvement? If so, the knee will lift on a straight arc-like pathway in space from its starting position to its lifted position. The pelvis will remain along the floor without nutation or counternutation.

1. Lie on your back with your knees bent, soles of the feet on the floor. Lengthen the spine along the floor and relax.
2. When ready, exhale and lift the thigh so that the shin raises to become parallel to the floor.
3. See if you can allow for deep folding in the inguinal area during the hip flexion. Become aware of any pelvic movement. It's fine to activate the hamstrings of the opposite leg (which remains with the sole of the foot on the floor) and to use the breath to promote initiation with the iliopsoas.
4. Notice whether the working leg moved directly upward or made a less than straight path. Was there rotation, either inward or outward? Was additional movement done in other parts of the body and if so, where did those parts move?
5. To examine differentiation or dissociation, ask: did the pelvis remain in its position, or did it move with the action of the thigh? For it to not be differentiating, it may have nutated or tilted so that the top of the sacrum moved down into the floor while the lower portion of the pelvis moved upward with the leg. It may have tilted sideways as well, or other actions may have occurred. Optimally, in this movement of the thigh lift, the femoral head would roll back and down in the hip joint as the distal end would trace a straight arc-like pathway directly upward toward the ceiling. If the

pelvis "went along with" the femur in some way, then there was not adequate differentiation of the two bones in the joint. This discovery would then be a topic for further exploration and work. The pathway made by the knee in space gives other information on what might be awry as well.

6. From the lifted position, then allow the leg to return to its start position of knee bent with sole of the foot returning to the floor. For this action, you may invite the hamstring to push the heel down into the floor (away from the ischium). Again, see what happened between the two bones of the hip. If there is adequate separation, the pelvic half will remain along the floor while the femur retraces its pathway back to the start.

7. This can then be done on the opposite side. Do not expect the pattern to necessarily be the same!

In coaching differentiation in this action, one wittingly or unwittingly uses space as the guide. When done with awareness of the pathway in space, the yoga therapist can observe, and communicate optimally. Keeping the sit bone reaching downward toward the heel along the floor, feeling the ball of the femur moving into the back of the joint space while the knee or distal end lifts upward on a diagonal pathway (forward, up), gives immense clarity to the mover. Hands-on guidance, demonstration, and verbal direction and redirection can accompany the specificity of the use of space for refining the movement pathway.

A quick note about orientation. In movement analysis there are two ways in which spatial movement can be oriented. It's good to stick with one or the other, or at least be clear about which one is in service so as not to be confusing. A map key or legend is an orientation to the map and its symbols. In space, there are two options for this. One is called the body key and the other the room key. Body key uses the body as the point of reference for the orientation in space. That is to say that the space being discussed is in relation to the body's dimensionality. Upward is always overhead for example. Room key uses the dimensions of the room as the reference point. If I am lying supine, upward in this case is toward the ceiling. If I lift my arm upward in the room key while lying supine, my hand will be in front of my chest, but it will be reaching upward in relation to the space of the room. If I remain in that position, but switch my orientation to body key, then my hand is now forward in space. This is because it is forward to my body with reference to it.

Support

When you think of support what comes to mind is likely strength and stability. I think of support as having enough stability in the right places in the body. Strength can be trained generally, but strength training can also be done through a range of motion that will be used in the actions and positions to be employed by the individual. This will involve both muscular strength and neuromuscular control.

Simple development of strength can be achieved through resistance training along the line of pull of a muscle or muscle group in question. Beyond this, functional action patterning of the body area can help develop and refine a more articulated use for greater aware control along a range. This type of training is often seen in dance, gymnastics, *yogasana* and *vinyasa*, and martial arts, in which the body's own weight is taken through greater and greater ranges of motion. Here we'll explore a simple action that requires support.

SOMATIC PRACTICE: Core support

This practice will progress in difficulty—please only do what you are comfortable doing with correct support. In this exploration, please keep your low back gently pressed to the floor. If you are unable to do so, then stop the exploration.

1. Lie supine with your knees bent and soles of your feet on the floor. Release your spine along the floor. To begin, lift your legs up off the floor so that the shins are more or less parallel to the floor.

2. As you slowly exhale, begin to lower one bent leg toward the floor, while keeping the low back pressed into the floor. Lower the leg only as far as you comfortably can with the low back pressed to the floor. To mediate the pull of the iliopsoas, use the transverse abdominals for this by squeezing toward your midline, narrowing throughout your torso. Also, activate your internal and external obliques by pulling the abdomen back toward your spine.

3. Then, as you begin to inhale, lift the leg back up to its starting position.

4. Repeat with the other leg.

5. If this was doable, then, to increase the training effect, repeat this action but this time allow the foot to land on the floor on exhale. Return on inhale. Remember, the low back needs to flow into the floor throughout the action. If you cannot maintain this, please stop, and go back to what was within your current capacity.

6. If step 5 was doable with support (which you can determine by seeing if you are maintaining the low back to the floor), this time extend the leg slightly so that the foot will land farther from your pelvis on the inhale and return on the exhale. Try the other side.

7. If step 6 is doable, see if you can do the action with each leg extending along the floor on inhale, returning on exhale.

You can see this is a progression that could be done to attain core support for these commonly used actions of the legs.

Organization

Organization refers to how the body is coordinated and orchestrated in action. Similar to a passage of music, movement also has phrases. And, like singing, the breath can play an important role in how the phrase of movement attempted is organized in time. Depending on the need, I work from local to global action training and then integrate that into the movement skill to be attained, such as kicking up smoothly into a handstand, pitching a no-hitter, or carrying a bag of groceries in from the car. Changing levels from low to middle to high and back often provides challenges to those seeking movement rehabilitation. The somatization below requires the use of a contralateral pattern, which in turn requires a reach of the upper limb. There are other possible reasons the movement could be inhibited and unsuccessful, such as a lack of differentiation in the hip or tightness in the low back. Still, it is a great exploration for understanding the importance that space has in accomplishing a movement successfully. If you do not reach into the space around the body in a spiraling path, the movement will be awkward and inefficient at best, impossible at worst. See what you think.

SOMATIC PRACTICE: Arm circle sit-up from Bartenieff's Basic Six

In this exploration you'll reach your lead arm (first the right, then the left) on a spiral pathway from the ground gradually upward to about shoulder height. This reach will allow you to roll to one side and come to a seated position keeping your knees off to that side.

1. Lie supine with your knees bent and soles of the feet on the floor. Now allow your knees to drop to the left side and your right arm to extend along the floor to your right slightly above your shoulder.
2. Now initiate from your right hand and reach it outward from your center as you draw an arc-like pathway along the floor (as best you can) over and across the top of your head, to your left, letting the body follow this action by rolling the torso to its left side.
3. Continue reaching outward and away from yourself as you reach along your left side, gradually reaching higher. Continue along the spiral pathway, allowing the arm reach to bring you to a sitting position with your knees off to your left, feet to the right, and right hand still reaching to right forward high in your body key.
4. When you're ready, trace the spiraled pathway in reverse and allow the body to return to the floor the way it came up to sitting.
5. Repeat this arm-circle sit-up on the other side.

You may not be able to sit up right away, and there could be various reasons for this. It may take some practice. However, the variable we're testing is the action of committing to *reaching in space* away from the body on the spiraling pathway. If you commit to that, the body's ability to organize into a contralateral pattern may indeed allow this movement to be light, free, easy, and fun!

EXPLORING INDIVIDUAL JOINTS AND SPACE

Yogis tend to have an intimate relationship with the spine. As our midline it is our bodily center around which we are organized to move in space. We contend with its curves and the attached weights of head, chest, and pelvis in the field of gravity. We have a host of body positions that arrange the limbs around it and change its orientation in space, with postures that move it in at least six common directions of extension, flexion, lateral flexion to each side, and rotation around its axis. These movements are often done as simultaneous actions of the whole spine, which means the entire spine moves as one thing.

Many of the issues of the spine come from its compression and imbalance in use over time. Reaching from each end of the spine and both ends at the same time can provide a postural remedy of sorts; not to eliminate its natural curves, but to bring space into the discs and to provide ligamentous support through the tautness of elongation of these companion tissues. It also can bring an aliveness of the entire spine into local actions. Reaching or pushing from either end or both ends of the spine can bring the whole spine into use.

A habitual action of turning to look when one's name is called can be localized to a twist at the neck. Patterning with spinal elongation upward and downward in space first, followed by initiation of movement from either end of the spine, can give the entire spine more support, which would then take pressure off the local joints of a body area.

SOMATIC PRACTICE: Elongation of the spine upward and downward for support

1. Sit in a comfortable position. Imagine someone calls your name (or actually have someone call your name) from behind your right shoulder.

2. Turn your head as usual and notice the activation of your spine and where its vertebrae are in space. See if you can "see" your spine in your body from tail to top of head, or, if you prefer, to the atlas bone just under your occiput.

3. Now gently elongate your spine by reaching the top of your head (or atlas) upward and the tip of your coccyx downward. Again, image someone calling your name from behind your right shoulder.

4. Start your head turn from the top of your spine (head or atlas) and follow through with the movement. What difference do you notice?

5. Try this again to the other side.

Another aspect of spinal concerns is lack of movement due to tightness of muscles from long-held postures, such as those needed to perform work sitting at a desk for long periods of time. The six movements of the spine mentioned above are a good start, especially for those new to yoga and those with a variety of movement-inhibiting restrictions along with little body awareness. Progressing even someone from this starting point into further articulation of the spine is possible with regular practice, accompanying visualization, hands-on coaching, giving clear spatial verbal directions, and demonstration.

Sequential spinal waves are perhaps the domain of pop icons and dance teams, but they can as well be an excellent way to identify tight and "offline" areas. Space plays a role here as the spinal waves take place as spinal movement in a plane. In a wave, each vertebra or larger bone such as the sacrum or occiput will tilt and move in a plane. For a sagittal spinal wave, that means the spine will inhabit space in the vertical and sagittal dimensions and not the horizontal one. The movement will take the bones in question forward and back. For a lateral wave the movement will take the bones side to side, and tilt them in the vertical plane.

SOMATIC PRACTICE: Spinal wave

These movements can be begun from the top or the bottom of the spine. The motion is serpentine and moves sequentially, which is to say, the movement travels from one bone to the next, not skipping or stopping anywhere along the entirety of the spine. In this exploration, become aware of the space in which the movement is happening.

Somatic practice: Bottom-up sagittal wave

1. Begin sitting in a chair or on the floor. If on the floor, arrange your legs so you are easily able to tilt your spine.

2. Initiate the movement by curling the tip of the tailbone forward. This will rock the top of the sacral bone back, with the lower part forward (counternutation). Allow this C-curve to travel all the way up your spine

to your skull. For this exploration we'll include the entire skull.

3. Once you feel the pattern has radiated all the way to the top of your head, begin the next action of reaching the tail slightly downward and back. Allow this action to reverberate through your entire spine to the top of your head as well. Allow movement to also take place freely in the rest of your body in response to this.

4. Once you have the gist of this, you can begin the initiation of the tailbone sooner. You can start it moving forward again while the prior movement is flowing through the thoracic or cervical area. See what timing works for you.

5. Once you have the pattern, please feel free to play with it, explore, and enjoy!

6. If you'd like to focus in on the space, get a good image of the spinal vertebrae. Feel each area, lumbar, thoracic, and cervical. Then once you have a fairly good somatic sense of the vertebrae in an area, begin the sagittal wave again but this time slow the movement down. See if you can track the action of one vertebra at a time. You don't need to study them all in one go. If there is an issue in an area, focus there, but don't lose sight of the whole as you do.

Somatic practice: Top-down sagittal wave

The top-down wave is performed in the same way, except that of course, the initiating body part, the head, is not weight bearing.

1. Initiate the movement by bringing the chin down then moving the head forward. Next, tilt the head back and reach the top of the head to back high. Allow the spine to lengthen slightly as you reach the head up and then bring the chin down again to repeat the entire movement.

2. See if you can allow the movement to travel through your entire spine. Allow movement to also take place freely in response to this in the rest of your body.

3. Take your time and see if you can find the various vertebrae and the space in which they are moving clearly. As above, see if you can track each vertebra as it moves as part of the chain.

4. Once you've done enough for you, stand, and take a walk. Notice what you notice.

Lateral spinal waves are also worth exploring. The movement is initiated with the head or tail moving off the one side, reaching away from the middle of the spine, and then crossing over to its opposite dimension: right to left, or left to right. When beginning at the bottom of the spine, weight shift through the pelvic halves is necessary. If you decide to explore this as well, notice how this exploration can inform gait patterning as well as reveal areas of tightness, lack of embodied awareness, and of course ineffective use of space for walking. If begun at the top with the head, please go slowly and maintain some control of the head. There are various important righting reactions and equilibrium responses at play when the head and eyes are no longer on the level.

When examining the use of space, good questions to ask are: Is the client or student able to move into the space the pattern requires? If not, why not? What is the cause? Is it an issue of differentiation, support, or organization? Or is it something else?

PROXIMAL JOINTS

Proximal joints present an interesting study of space for the body. The hip and shoulder joints are ball and socket joints, so theoretically they should be easy to map spatially with the femur or humerus distal end's abilities to circumduct in a large portion of the kinesphere around its joint socket. Looking for range of motion at these joints, however, when focused on functional use, provides information on unique characteristics that can benefit from clarity of movement in space.

SOMATIC PRACTICE: Hip circumduction

1. Begin lying supine with your knees bent and soles of the feet on the floor.
2. Allow the right leg to extend upward into the air above the hip. You can place the other shin on a raised support to help support your low back in this position or push slightly into the floor with the left foot to help you stabilize.
3. Leading with your right foot, or, if you prefer, your knee, draw a very small circle in the air. The circle should exist mainly in the horizontal plane.
4. Now begin to enlarge the circle, slowly tracing an enlarging circle. Allow its size to grow as much as you like as long as you can maintain the starting body position without strain. Bring your leg down and rest.
5. When you are ready, repeat the circling in the opposite direction. Bring the leg down and rest. What do you notice?
6. Now roll to your left side with the knees bent and arms and head arranged in a way that is comfortable to you.
7. Turn your right leg out (laterally rotate it in the hip), bend the knee and place the foot on the floor in front of you or place it on the lower shin. Raise your knee and explore the movement possible here while remaining in this side-lying position. Allow the leg to rotate medially and notice the difference in the ease and spatial range as you do. Rest.
8. Turn to the other side and explore with the left leg as above. Rest.

What did you notice about your spatial ranges for each femur and leg in both of these positions?

SOMATIC PRACTICE: Shoulder circumduction

1. Lie on your left side with the knees bent and arms and head arranged in a way that is comfortable to you. Lift your top arm so the arm is stacked above your shoulder socket.
2. Begin drawing a very small circle in the air with your hand. The circle should exist mainly in the horizontal plane.
3. Now begin to enlarge the circle, slowly tracing an enlarging circle. Allow its size to grow as much as you like as long as you can maintain the starting position without strain. Bring your arm down and rest.
4. When you are ready, repeat the circling in the opposite direction. Bring the arm down and rest.
5. Turn to your other side and repeat the exploration. What do you notice?

Below are two applications of spatial awareness in relation to the proximal joints of shoulders and hips that demonstrate the value of spatial awareness and the ability of not only sensing but observing and articulating this awareness in improving movement efficiency.

SOMATIC PRACTICE: Clock-face weight shift

This exploration can be helpful in patterning efficient dynamic alignment of the legs in weight shift, which is basically any stepping, running, hopping, or jumping movement. Careful practice, with attention to where the body parts are and how they relate to one another in space, can develop into patterning for optimal use.

Prior to beginning this exploration, please be aware of three hip positions: parallel, which is to keep the feet pointing directly forward; turned out from the hip with the toes out and heels close, Charlie Chaplin style; and turned in from the hip, with the toes inward and heels outward. Please note I'm calling these hip positions in that you will rotate the entire leg from the hip to achieve them.

1. Stand and imagine the face of a clock painted on the floor with the numbers surrounding you. You are standing in the middle where the clock's arms originate. The numbers are close enough for you to step on if taking a normal-sized step in any direction.

2. Bend your knees slightly and feel the soles of your feet. Imagine the shape of a triangle from the center of the heel to the knuckle of the large toe to the knuckles between your fourth and fifth toe on the sole of each foot. Image and feel this shape and place your weight as evenly as you can on each corner of the triangle.

3. Now pay attention to your pelvic floor. Draw an imaginary line, like the path a batter runs on a baseball diamond, from your pubic symphysis to the right ischial tuberosity, to the tip of your coccyx and to your left ischial tuberosity. Use an image of the pelvic floor and its bony landmarks to help locate these points as you like.

4. From a slightly bent knee position, step forward to twelve o'clock. While doing so, feel the tailbone shift over the heel point and the pubis shift over the knuckle of the large toe. Allow the sit bone on that side to center over the knuckles between the fourth and fifth toes on that side.

5. Then shift back to the foot that remained in the starting place. While doing so, again feel the tailbone shift over the heel point and the pubis shift over the knuckle of the large toe. Allow the sit bone on that side to center over the knuckles between the fourth and fifth toes on that side as you shift back to place. This is the basic maneuver; track this relationship during weight shift.

6. Once you feel you have the basic sense of it, then begin to step to different numbers of the clock while keeping your pelvis mainly forward facing. Of course, you don't need to step to the exact whole numbers on the clock, you can step between them if you prefer—step to 9:42 if you like! The idea is to shift your weight into different spaces around you while keeping good dynamic leg alignment using the relationship of these two body areas.

7. When you are ready and have got a good sense of the alignment with the weight shifts, please try the stepping again but now with the hips turned out, and turned in. Feel free to mix them up: turned out, turned in, parallel, but keep the

alignment in place for the weight transfer throughout.

8. As a bonus, once you can make the weight shifts in all directions with all three hip positions, then take a few steps in each direction, and then return to the center. Also vary the timing and finally the level, moving lower to higher while keeping correct dynamic alignment of the legs.

This is a good way to develop skill in weight transference while being aware of the directional changes of the body in space. This could easily develop into more stylized actions like short dance, or martial arts movement sequences if arms and torso movements are added.

SCAPULOHUMERAL RHYTHM

Sooner or later, exploring the movement potential of the shoulder joint brings us to the combined action of the shoulder girdle bones of the clavicle or collarbone, the scapula or shoulder blade, and the humerus or upper arm bone. Taking the arm overhead in yoga is a common practice. Feeling the correct functioning of the movement of the bones of the shoulder girdle in this action can be understood by using space to describe what is going on. For this exploration we'll take the arm generally out to the side in what is known as the scapular plane. From being at the side of the body, the arm will move on a forward diagonal pathway: right forward low to middle to high, and, on the other side, from left forward low to middle to high.

The scapulohumeral rhythm is a synchronized movement, but for the purpose of assessing

spatial clarity we'll break the movement down into a few steps. Once abducting the arm through the scapular plane is explored, go on to flex the shoulder, bringing it forward and up. Lift it in other pathways to further explore the actions and relationships of these bones in movement.

Before you begin the practice below, find a good picture of the shoulder girdle bones from the side so you can see the glenoid fossa or socket as well as the scapula bone itself. Note that the shape of the scapula is curved to follow the curve of the ribs. If we follow a line from the inner edge of the shoulder blade out through the shoulder socket, we see the socket is angled forward at around 30 degrees. This line is called the scapular plane. What adjustment would need to be made in the joint or in the placement of the scapula to raise the arm directly to the side?

SOMATIC PRACTICE: Scapulohumeral rhythm

1. Begin standing. Elevating the humerus to slightly below the shoulder level is our first step.

2. Explore raising your arm to the forward diagonal direction along the scapular plane. Notice any sense of unimpeded ease. Now, without changing the position of your scapula, try raising your arm

directly to the side. What difference, if any, do you notice?

3. Looking again at the lateral view of the shoulder blade, you'll see the acromion and coracoid processes extend outward above the socket (glenoid fossa). Other tissues layered onto this form a ledge of sorts above the humerus bone. At the

top of the humerus is its round head, which fits into the socket of the scapula. On the outer part of the humerus is a protuberance called the greater tubercle. When abducting the humerus to the side, the greater tubercle will run into the ledge, blocking the movement. Continuing to push through this could cause an impingement of sensitive tissues in the subacromial space, especially if scapular movement is inhibited in some way. The solution is to externally rotate the arm in order to further abduct it. This is taking the tubercle back in space and then allowing the elbow to move higher. Explore externally rotating the greater tubercle of your humerus moving backward in space to allow for more clearance as you lift the arms to the sides.

4. Take some time to explore medially and laterally rotating your humerus and lifting your arms to the front, sides, and on various trajectories within your comfortable capacity. This is the second step of scapulohumeral rhythm, externally rotating the humerus to further abduct the arm.

5. The next step is to sense the upward rotation of the scapula as the arm continues upward. For the arm to continue higher on its pathway without inhibition, the inner upper corner of the scapula will move downward while its lower tip moves laterally—this being the action of its rotation. If you have another person present, ask them to do this while you place your hands over their scapula to feel this movement. This movement usually doesn't take place until after about the first 30 degrees of humeral elevation. Beyond that point the shoulder blade will come along with the arm, allowing you then to bring the arm all the way overhead.

6. The next action we're isolating is called the posterior tilt of the scapula and it is a very important aspect when working with older adults and folks who sit at desks and type for long periods. This is because upper crossed syndrome, a muscular imbalance, often results from long-term embodiment of the common head-forward, upper-back-rounded position of modern living. The scapula in its natural position on the back with the arm hanging at the side conforms to the contour of the ribs, which curve forward at the top. The top of the scapula follows this curve with its upper portion tilting forward. As the arm abducts, the action of the scapula during the upper part of the arm's journey tilts in the opposite direction, with the top tilting backward in space. In a lot of people, for a lot of reasons, this movement is minimal, so it is something to look for, sense, and palpate as possible. This is also called scapular external rotation.

As you explore you may decide to attend to companionate clavicular, thoracic, or other supportive movement. Not only isolating these actions when looking at shoulder function, but observing where the bones are moving in space, gives important insight into what specific strategies can be put into place to improve movement function.

HEAD, NECK, AND JAW RHYTHMS

In terms of body use, I think of rhythms as coordinating parts with movement function the unifying factor. When we're born, our spine is curved like the letter "C." As we move and gain motor control, we may find ourselves prone, on our tummies. As we lift our heads to see what is happening around us, the cervical curve is formed. The joint at the base of the skull is called the atlanto-occipital joint. The top vertebra, the atlas, named for the Greek Titan who was defeated by Zeus and so destined to carry the weight of the world on his neck, does not have a posterior process. The occipital bone at the base of the skull has two small protuberances, called the occipital condyles, that sit at either side of its foramen magnum. Fortunately the atlas has two small indentations in which these little knobs fit, to help balance the head on the top of the serpentine spine.

This joint is an important one in terms of head position and movement, but it only allows for forward and down, and backward and up, nodding of the head. To turn the head to the side, we need to go one vertebra down to the axis. This vertebra has a posterior spinous process and a dens, which is a small vertical spike around which the atlas revolves. Basically, you nod yes from your atlanto-occipital joint, and shake your head no from the atlanto-axial joint.

The temporo-mandibular joints (TMJ) are located between the jawbone (mandible) and temporal bones on the side of the skull. Their motion is varied and complex as they slide and rotate just in front of each ear. The muscles of these joints allow the mandible to move up and down, side to side, and forward and back, with each side working independently. Free well-coordinated movements of chewing, talking, yawning, and swallowing and the like all take place here, and problems can occur when imbalance and tension in these areas create misalignment in position and action.

The relationships between the movements of the head, jaw, hyoid, and spine in the region of the neck are profound and complex. Sucking, swallowing, head righting, balance, and equilibrium responses all involve this area, and the motion of these two joints can play a large role. In fact, the movement of one joint is always in relation to other joints in the body. Spatial awareness, a refined sensing of where each part is located, and the *direction* it is moving can go far in remedial work and refinement of action, especially in a body area of such structural delicacy and intricate movement.

SOMATIC PRACTICE: AOJ–AAJ–TMJ

1. Take your two middle fingers and find the ridge of the base of your skull in the back of your head. Trace this to the midline and see if you can find the indentation under which the atlas bone is located. See if you can feel and imagine where the base of the skull and the very top of the spine meet at the atlanto-occipital joint. Initiate a very small nod of the head, moving it up and down from this place of awareness. You may wish to close your eyes for this. Notice any movement at the temporo-mandibular joint.

2. Then take your fingers a little lower and see if you can palpate the spinous process of the axis bone. See if you can feel and imagine the atlanto-axis joint (AAJ) as you make a tiny side-to-side turn of your head from this joint. You may wish to close your eyes for this. Notice any movement at the temporo-mandibular joint.

3. To locate your temporo-mandibular joint, place your index fingers just in front of your ears. Open and close your jaw as if chewing a few times. See if you can feel the condylar process of the jawbone moving on an arc-like pathway, diagonally forward and down, and back and up. Trace

the edges of the bone down to the "cor-ner" or angle of the manubrium. See what other movements are possible. Notice any movement at the atlanto-occipital joint as you do so.

4. Sit in front of a desk or table and place your elbows on it. Place your jaw on your hands as you might when resting your head on your hand to listen and stabilize the jaw. Now move the skull with the jaw remaining stationary. Notice the resulting movement of your skull in space. Where does it move?

5. Now tilt your head into your hands like you might do when you have a headache. Stabilizing the head in this way move your jaw. Now let your head come up onto your spine and yawn, speak, chew, or drink something, and notice the relationship of these joints.

6. One more thing: eat something like an apple or a juicy orange, or sip some soup from a large spoon so that your mouth has to shape and reach and gather around the objects and fluids. Notice the coordinated movement in these joints.

Sucking and swallowing actions involve an orchestration of these joints as well. An infant able to nurse at the breast will bring the mother's nipple well into its mouth. Singing and chanting vowel sounds will mirror this shaping of the softer tissues involved as well as orchestrate the smooth coordinated movement of these joints. Moving down the neck and including the hyoid bone and the vocal diaphragm is rich territory worthy of further investigation. Solutions to long-held problems can be discovered when working somatically. Observation and exploration are key. Experientially noticing, then inhabiting, then carefully repatterning tissues for greater functional use, and all that comes with such change, is within the domain of yoga therapy.

OVERALL USE OF THE BODY IN SPACE: GLOBAL JOINT USE

In the exploration above we zoomed in on a particular body area and its movement capacity with awareness. We can also use an astute awareness of space to benefit the overall use of the entire body, which includes a global awareness of the joints. The next somatization is derived from my experience of the Alexander Technique as taught by my Alexander teacher, Aileen Crow. Aileen was a master movement therapist with a wide range of somatic training and was someone with whom I studied and was mentored by for many decades. I include this somatization with the note that the version I'm sharing is not a sanctioned one but is the way I've been using what was passed to me from Aileen.

F. M. Alexander was a Shakespearean orator who developed laryngitis while he was performing. Finding no medical explanation, he took matters into his own hands and studied the way he moved as he spoke by looking closely at himself in a mirror. Detecting subtle muscular tension from tilting his head back and down (chin up), he noted this depressed his larynx. He eventually developed an entire technique that began with the direction to release the head "forward and up" (chin down). He called this action of releasing the back of the head upward and the jaw slightly downward the primary control. From his initial discoveries he developed a hands-on technique that teaches the student to use the body with more whole-body integration, ease, freedom, and efficiency.

SOMATIC PRACTICE: Releasing into expansion somatization

The directions are given with the overall intention of releasing unnecessary tension thus allowing each area of the body to occupy its own space. This then brings greater ease, better alignment, and freer and fuller movement. The body expands in space due to yielding or relaxing into it, not by activating with effort. This is a skill that can be learned for greater ease of use throughout the body. The practice can be done sitting or standing. The directions given below are for a seated position. They should be given with a pause after each one, so the person practicing may have time to sense and achieve the direction.

1. Allow the head to release forward and up, so you can...
2. allow the spine to lengthen and the back to widen
3. allow the ischial tuberosities to release into the chair (or if standing to drop downward)
4. allow the knees to release forward (only if sitting)
5. allow the feet to release into the floor.

This sequence of directions allows the body to take up its rightful space, reduces overall tension, encourages alignment, and permits the head freedom to lead movement.

EXPLORING REACH SPACE AND KINETIC CHAINS

So far, we've been exploring use of space in terms of particular directions and how awareness of where body parts are in space, and how they're orchestrated with spatial clarity, can help repatterning improved movement function. This can also be addressed spatially in a more general way, inviting the client to invest more in space, taking up more of it, or condensing its use—each for a specific beneficial purpose in another useful more global approach.

A kinesphere is the sphere around the body that can be reached easily without stepping off one's place. Place can be thought of like a base in baseball that the base runner must at least keep one foot on. The kinesphere, or movement sphere, is also referred to as one's reach space. Movement taking place close to the body is considered movement in near reach. Movement taking place at the periphery of the kinesphere is in far reach, and movement between these takes place in middle reach. We can keep our actions close in near reach, say as you would when cuddling an infant. You likely use middle reach when doing deskwork, and far reach when washing a large-paned window. Mostly we vary our space, gesturing closer and farther based on what we're doing.

The kinetic chain is a concept used to consider movement as it sequences through the body. Joints, muscles, fascia, and nerve impulses all come into play in producing smooth, effective, and efficient movement. How do we know if a movement is effective? It achieves its goal. It is efficient if it doesn't need to rely on compensatory patterning that asks the body to move in ways that, in the long term, or sometimes in the immediate, cause pain and injury.

In movement analysis we can look at the pathway of movement through the body as well as the pathway of movement of the body in space. Close examination of both will yield vital information on how the body is compensating for a weakness or lack of support, too much binding of tissues or muscular tension, or faulty neuromuscular sequencing and misalignment.

Kinetic chains are ways of considering how

the movement flows through the body, especially the limbs. The idea of observing the efficiency of effect from where the movement begins or initiates and how it sequences from one part to the next adjacent part came from engineering—which makes total sense. Kinetic chains are grouped into two types: closed and open. A closed kinetic chain is performed when the distal end of a limb is fixed (closed) against an immovable surface, resulting in the proximal portions moving. The resistance felt through that limb produces the chain of movement. Cat-Cow on all fours is an example from *yogasana* practice. This has a stabilizing effect and promotes the interdependence of several parts of the body. These features can be considered for use in designing therapeutic practices.

An open kinetic chain is performed when the distal end of a limb is free to move in space. Reaching an arm out to the side from Cat or Table Pose is an example. This type of movement often singles out a muscle or muscle group. This feature of open chain flow can be considered for use in designing therapeutic practices as well.

In my experience, closed chain movements take us into relation with gravity and involve push patterns, while open chain movements involve reaching into and propulsion into space—of either our body as in a leap or a swing, or an object in a throw or a toss. In terms of self and other, they both can be ways in which we receive; I can lower myself into gravity as well as catch a throw or receive something passed to me.

SOMATIC PRACTICE: Reach space and kinetic chains

For this practice you will need a partner and a ball you can comfortably catch with your bare hands. If you and your partner are not skilled in "playing catch" please toss the ball underhand and allow it to bounce once or twice before catching it. You can do this alone, but the sense of kinetic chains will not be nearly as pronounced because you will be investing in much less space, unless you can work in a large space outdoors and are willing to bounce the ball hard and run after it!

1. Stand a comfortable distance from your partner and toss the ball to them. Throwing is usually done overhand, which means that the ball is released with the palm and fingers above it. A toss is done underhand, with the ball leaving the palm of the hand underneath it.

2. As you toss or throw, notice your movement phrasing as you prepare, throw, and then recuperate after releasing the ball.

3. As you catch the ball, notice your movement phrasing as you prepare, catch, and then recuperate after receiving the ball.

4. Now notice the space you use as you both throw and then catch. Do you come from the center outward, do you change your facing? Do you step forward or side? What do you do spatially to support your goal of throwing and catching the ball?

5. Try throwing by beginning with awareness of your physical center, then move from near through middle to far reach. Try catching by being aware of the space outside of your kinesphere, then contact the ball through far, then middle, then near reach.

6. Now notice your lower body and its contact with the earth as you "load and cock" your arm to throw. Can you feel the force or power that comes from your stance?

7. Now notice your upper body, especially your throwing arm, as you wind up to throw and then release the ball. Do you

sense the movement radiating outward sequentially through your limb?

8. Do the same while catching; notice your arm or arms as they receive the ball responding to its speed and direction.

Notice your legs (and the rest of your body) as you accommodate the ball coming into your kinesphere. Notice how you adapt to get a hold of it and control the ball's motion.

Issues of giving and receiving, separating from other and differentiating, as well as sequencing with awareness of all the parts involved, arise from working with the kinetic chains in relation to reach space pathways from near-to-far and far-to-near. Practicing favorite *vinyasa* sequences can also be a great place to explore these concepts.

Even better would be to make up new sequences that involve a variety of spatial uses that benefit specific joints, muscle imbalances, and neuromuscular patterns according to identified specific needs.

CHAPTER 5

Embodying Body Organization

When body parts move in coordination, each with distinct and clear spatial pathways and precise movement quality, movement is considered well articulated. This is like speech, when a point is well expressed, and an argument is well built so that comprehension is clear. In movement the goal is effective action with minimal energy wasted and negligible wear and tear.

After considering how the body is organized to move in space, it's useful to look at movement phrasing in time. Like a sentence or passage of music, a movement can be considered to have a preparation, a beginning, main action, follow-through, and recovery, or more simply a preparation, action, and recovery. You might wonder how this is useful in movement efficiency. The answer is that the timing of the movement is clarified by an understanding of phrasing. In yoga this can often be coordinated well by the breath. In *vinyasa* movement, at times a single action like raising the arms overhead is done with an inhale. Then the reverse, lower the arms, is done on the exhale. One might consider this a singular phrase consisting of one breath cycle. In designing therapeutic *vinyasa*, the ratio of the breath to the timing of the movement can be altered. This simple phrase could be altered in timing so that the arm movement could be slowed enough so the arms could raise and lower all on the inhalation, and again on the exhalation, and so forth. The timing of the movement would be designed according to the goal for the practice. In whatever case, the phrase of movement can be felt and understood as a singular statement.

GREATER ARTICULATION IN MOVEMENT SEQUENCING THROUGH INITIATION AND PART LEADING

Initiation, as it sounds, is the start of the movement phrase. A preparation could occur prior to it in which the identifiable movement may not have yet begun but there is a slight qualitative moment of shift into readiness to act. It is a moment in pre-motor focus in which the neuromuscular system, you might say, loads the execution into its system. I have found this to be the point of no return for repatterning and that to make a change in the execution of a movement I must give new information to the body *prior* to the preparation.

What happens in movement after the initiation is the organized execution of the movement phrase or phrases as planned. This is done as the moving person (mover) pays attention (or doesn't) to the feedback perceived as during execution. In movement analysis this is called sequencing; it is how the movement phrase unfolds. More specifically, successive movement is movement that unfolds in a step-by-step sequence of adjacent actions.

Once the movement is initiated and has begun, the part of the body where the movement was initiated, i.e., where it began, can continue to lead the movement, or a different part can take over the lead. Whatever body part is leading the movement is considered the part leading. This may require a new initiation, or it may be part of the initial motor plan. Movement phrasing can be complex and can give movement its "signature" characteristics, such as can be seen the ways people enact the same movement but give it different nuance in performance. There of course are other variables as well!

SOMATIC PRACTICE: Initiation and successive sequencing of spinal rotation

1. Side-sit with your knees bent to the left side with both feet going toward the right side of your body. Spread your legs slightly so that you have a wide enough base between your front and back hips to sit upright. If you are unable to sit upright in this position, you may wish to get a block or rolled blanket to place under your supporting hip.

2. Begin with your weight forward in the front hip and spiral your spine gently to the left.

3. Initiate a movement phrase by shifting your weight to the back hip, leading down and back with the right sit bone.

4. Continue with shifting more and more of your weight gradually into the back pelvic half while you rotate successively up your spine, vertebra by vertebra, to the right, with the very last part of the phrase being your head turning due to the swivel of the atlanto-axial joint.

5. Now initiate a return or retrograde movement by shifting your weight to the front of your left hip, leading down and forward with the left sit bone.

6. Continue shifting more and more of your weight gradually into the front pelvic half while you rotate successively up your spine, vertebra by vertebra, to the left, with the very last part of the phrase being your head turning due to the swivel of the atlanto-axial joint.

7. Once you have this movement in your body, decide how you wish to coordinate your breath with it; this will affect the tempo of your movement.

8. If you're inclined, repeat this exploration initiating from the turn of your head, letting it sequence downward through your body and then upward.

You may wish to further investigate what could happen to the movement if, while you are turning, you add an additional element like having the lead arm take over as the part leading. Such complex movements are part of our everyday movement life if we interact with others in movement in space like in sports and similar responsive activities.

INITIATION, PART LEADING, AND SEQUENCING IN ANALYSIS OF MOVEMENT EFFICIENCY

Movements from the Bartenieff Fundamentals Basic Six are an excellent way to observe articulation through initiation, part leading, and sequencing in movement phrasing. Above we explored successive movement that traveled throughout the body using a body part at one end of the torso as the point of initiation.

Simultaneous movement is a good choice when we wish to use considerable force in an action, or when we propel ourselves from more than one body area or limb. It is valuable in many other ways as well. The exploration below uses the pelvic forward shift movement from the Basic Six. It is a movement that can be seen when one stands from a seated position, shifting weight evenly onto both legs. It can also be seen when one jumps off the feet and lands on both. The standing long jump, in which both feet leave the ground and land together, is an example of this. The pelvic forward shift is like the archetype of this homologous pattern and is a strengthening movement of stability and power.

SOMATIC PRACTICE: Pelvic forward shift

1. Lie supine with your knees bent and the soles of the feet on the floor, knees upward to the ceiling.
2. Exhale and press downward on the feet, engaging the hamstrings while at the same time lifting the pelvis straight upward. The tailbone may be actively curled slightly under as part of the simultaneous initiating and movement off all of these parts at one time.
3. See if your pelvis moved evenly upward, without tilting in any direction or favoritism shown to one side or one leg. Then slowly inhale to lower the pelvis again to the floor.
4. Repeat several more times as you like.

See if you're able to do this movement without a lot of other activation going on. Are you able to clearly move the pelvis forward (body key) in space with both hips even? If you like, practice the movement until you've taken anything extraneous out of it. Find the best way or ways to use your breath until you're able to activate a truly simultaneous movement phrase orchestrating all the functional body areas with ease.

WHOLE-BODY ORGANIZATION IN MOVEMENT SOMATIZATION

In looking at rehabilitation and re-facilitation of movement function we work with differentiation, support, and organization of the body as three categories of focus that help us discern the area of work. At times there may be overlap to the point that the original issue—whether it be injury, weakness causing a misalignment over time, or lack of motor coordination—becomes blurred. Still, in seeking a course of remedy, much of what we do is to zoom in to discern a precise area of work, then proceed to work in an articulate manner.

At times, however, this doesn't produce the results anticipated. It then may be time to pull the lens back to a wide-angle view and look less precisely and particularly, instead observing globally and wholly.

This approach to whole-body organization came to me over many years. And while I respect, have studied, and at times teach from more articulated vocabularies of somatic work, I use these two patterns of organization as my first, most general lens. When I look at the whole body, I look at the sculptural form made in space, i.e., what the body shape looks like. I look at what appears to be the center of this form. I'm looking at whether the body is: (1) organized around the navel center or (2) organized around the midline. I had early experiences of both whole-body patterns becoming an integral part of my movement life. To illustrate, I'll share a personal experience of both.

I grew up a reluctant athlete until I found dance—then it all made sense. My mother was a physical education teacher who would, on occasion, bring home new equipment to try out for her well-loved classes. One of these was the tumbling belt. It's a device worn around the hips or waist with two ropes attached by swivels to each side. It's used to assist tumblers in handsprings, flips, and other stunts of this nature. The "spotters" run alongside the tumbler, and at the crucial moment assist by hoisting the tumbler's center of weight in the right direction. This gives the tumbler a sense of where their body center should go in space, and to some degree how fast it needs to get there, to succeed in the movement attempted. Of course a lot of things must work together to achieve something like a back flip, including the preceding round-off and back handspring that help to increase momentum. During my elementary school years I'd not the inclination nor the bravery commensurate to the task, yet found myself strapped in and hoisted through the air in my backyard as part of my mother's trial runs with new equipment. I have a distinct recollection of my mother remarking

that I didn't know where my center was in space. This caused me to double down and lead with my head, which of course made the whole thing worse.

I later discovered that I did in fact know how to track my center of gravity. This was while spinning on a rope hung on a large black walnut tree. I would sit on the huge knot at the end of the rope and walk along the side of the tree to wind the rope around it. Then I'd push off to see how many spins I could get in while the rope made a huge arcing pathway around the tree as it unwound and rewound around the tree in the opposite direction. I mastered this in the horizontal plane by drawing all the parts of my body in toward my center and tracking the revolutions through my kinesthetic sense. The flip I'd failed to master was in the sagittal plane. I somehow eventually put together that this knowing where I was in space could be applied to the handsprings and flips at which I'd earlier failed, by switching my orientation to the planes.

Organizing around my midline was more of a conscious practice I was taught to do. I'd been studying yoga at the YMCA as a child. My teacher, Margaret Hill, had instructed me in the meditative seated position with head, neck, and torso aligned in the vertical dimension. I believe this gave me an advantage in archery, at which I was very good, and in balancing—another strength. As demonstrated during my tumbling belt encounter, I knew my head atop was an important middle division, but alas that was not the kind of organization I needed to learn handsprings and flips.

Much later I learned about the primitive reflexes, righting reactions, and equilibrium responses, that certainly come into play when learning how to do a flip! My study of these automatic actions was not as isolated checkpoints but as building blocks that allow the body to organize pathways of movement to greater and greater movement facility. This approach came from

Bonnie Bainbridge Cohen's Body-Mind Centering®. It presented, among many other marvelous things, a way to work with movement repatterning involving the whole body through unifying patterns Bonnie now calls the Basic Neurocellular Patterns. The patterns are developmental in that they represent stages gone through, yet the work acknowledges each person's own unique relationship to the patterns. Here development may be, but is not necessarily, linear. Some stages may have more or less investment experientially so that movement strengths and weaknesses may accrue. Yet the patterns are big enough to underlie and inform a person's entire movement repertoire.

In addition, this work is not layered onto the body as imagery sometimes can be. Rather, it comes from deep within the body's neurological system, using the reflexes, right reactions, and equilibrium responses as a sort of alphabet of movement, as Bonnie has called it in *Sensing, Feeling, and Action* (2012), that provide pathways for movement patterning. My experience is that these pathways act as the superhighways of organization when we tap into them. They provide a lightness, a clarity, and ease that can be capitalized on.

And because this somatic work takes place in and through the body, and these patterns come into play during our early, preverbal development, deep psychomotor content may arise, appearing as vague emotions or sensations and movement disorganization. These experiences lay down our neural platform for establishing movement patterns and preferences. These in tern have bearing on our modes of communication, learning, and embodied sense of agency.

The Basic Neurocellular Patterns are separated into two groups that relate well to my center and midline organizational patterns. They are pre-vertebrate and vertebrate patterns that relate to patterns used by various species. Even though Haeckel's theory of recapitulation, in which "ontogeny recapitulates phylogeny," has been debunked, Cohen's work presents fascinating similarities in functional movement organization between various species' movement and that of humans throughout the stages of development.

The early species the Basic Neurocellular Patterns mirror in human movement development are classified as pre-vertebrates—think jellyfish and starfish. The movement emanating from these mostly acquatic creatures is flowing, undulatory, and streaming. They remind me of the squirming movements of a newborn, adapting to the use of their digestive system, and the wavelike motions I remember during pregnancy that would pass across my abdomen. These patterns are useful in water or possibly when flying through the air but are not directly helpful in locomotion on land when skeletal support is a more optimal way to get around. Body-Mind Centering® currently identifies the pre-vertebrate patterns as: vibration, cellular breathing, sponging, pulsation, navel radiation, mouthing, and prespinal. I studied this work prior to the explication of vibration, sponging, and pulsation, although I believe elements of these were embedded in the progression. Because I don't have a long-term experiential basis in my own body for these patterns, I'll not discuss them here. I will briefly discuss my understanding of these patterns as whole body organizing experiences. The School for Body-Mind Centering® has many programs and video resources available if you'd like to go more deeply into this rich and profound material.

FOUR SELECTED PRE-VERTEBRATE PATTERNS

Cellular breathing

Cellular breathing refers to the activity of cells to nourish and expel. This life-sustaining act reflects "The Big In and the Big Out" of the universal pulse of *brahmana* and *langhana* (expanding and condensing). There is also an element of autonomous intelligence in that the cell membrane discerns what will pass through it and in what amounts.

Whether we can feel this happening or not within our bodies, focusing on the process and noticing areas in which our tissues feel more enlivened compared to those that do not, identifying areas in need of tonification or possessing too much stimulation, can be a body awareness technique leading to deep rest, support, and healing. In the vocabulary of yoga practice, awareness is a powerful tool. Yoga theory proposes that the subtle level is more potent than the gross. As the adage goes, "Prana flows where the mind goes."

As a whole-body pattern, to me cellular breathing is that of a form organized around a central nucleus, with a fluid streaming base for internal and sometimes external movement. My experience of cellular breathing is that my cells and tissues are an intelligent functioning collective that maintains its individual conditions for optimal wellness, having an overall effect. When I focus on cellular function, I imagine I tap into the innate intelligence of life processes always going on within my body.

Navel radiation

Navel radiation has the sense of center and periphery, with ebb and flow from center to edge and back underlying. In my experience, the navel radiation pattern includes lines radiating from center to points on the periphery. With differentiation into lines, forces of external movement can be generated. We see this pattern in starfish (echinoderm) living in water and moving using a pattern of radial symmetry with the control center in the middle of its many limbs. In our early in utero development we embody this organization as a fluid-surrounded fetus connected to source through the umbilical cord at our navel. In this pattern, our head, two arms, two legs, and tail (coccyx) are equal in their ability to extend simultaneously into the space around and condense or draw into center in one synchronized action. This is the pattern I do not think I had well developed (even though I needed it) when I was strapped into that tumbling belt!

Mouthing

Mouthing and prespinal patterns differentiate the head-limb as unique in its importance. In humans, several important senses congregate in the head, rather than being distributed on the ends of limbs like the photoreceptors of a starfish. We do, however, retain an abundance of nerve endings on our non-head limbs of hands and feet.

The mouthing pattern begins in utero and, for a newborn, eating and digesting are the main waking occupations. The oral rooting reflex starts the process of movement in search of the nipple. Further movement snaking the milk through the digestive tract from mouth to anus ensues. And it is of a soft wiggling, pushing, and wormlike nature, which is what the digestive tube itself resembles. Having quiet settled time for nursing gives the infant a way to organize itself around these deep, whole-body patterns.

Prespinal

This digestive action is our first throughline from top to bottom around our vertical axis. To me it is the whisper of the pattern I identified as midline. Body-Mind Centering® identifies the prespinal pattern as an outgrowth of mouthing-based organization. But whereas mouthing is organized by the gut tube, the prespinal pattern is oriented around an embryonic axis called the notochord. In early fetal development, human beings pass through a stage in which the notochord runs along the vertical axis. The brain and spinal cord develop posteriorly while the gut tube develops anteriorly. Eventually the notochord disappears, with a trace element of it seen in the fluid-filled intervertebral discs of the spine. Before it does, however, it provides the scaffolding to anchor the spine, and muscular and nervous system tissues developing along the spinal cord. Yet the sense of midline, or "soft spine" as I've heard it called, remains. We see this gentle movement as the soft undulations of traditional dances of the South Pacific and in other dance forms.

SOMATIC PRACTICE: Organization around the center

Part 1

1. Lie comfortably on your back and close your eyes. You may want a small cushion under your knees or head. Allow your body to relax into the field of gravity. Feel the skin that envelops the entire body. Take a moment to notice the skin all around the perimeter of your body.

2. Now bring your attention to the breath. Notice the movement that happens in the body as you breathe. Notice the movements near where you are breathing in and out, and notice the subtle movements farther away from this. Become aware that your entire physical body is made up of many, many cells. These cells are of different types, different tribes with different missions, yet they are all your body's cells. They are different tissues, different teams of cells working together for a common aim, and they are all breathing. They each take in nutrients and oxygen, burning the nutrients in the fire of cellular *agni*, thus generating energy. Then they expel waste.

3. From the metabolic fire in the cell's mitochondrial "furnace," our eating and breathing match up and transform into the energy we use to live. The cells live if this process goes well and is balanced. We, as a collective of cells of different tribes, live less well if this process does not go well in different areas and tribes. The cells also exhale, they expel waste back out through their cell walls, back into the bloodstream. Through their cell wall, which is a smart membrane, the cells are breathing. Imagine, if you like, that they are minutely expanding from their center and they are minutely contracting toward their center. They are breathing. Feel the whole body, alive, and breathing on the cellular level. Feel the lungs breathing on the external whole-organism level too. Can you feel how these two processes support one another?

Part 2

4. Now pay attention to your navel center, where your umbilical cord once was, where you were attached to nourishment, and the point around which your movements were oriented.

5. Notice your skin, all around your body, enveloping the other aspects of your body, a membrane, a smart sensitive container. Your nervous system arises out of the same tissue that becomes your skin. Your innermost and your outermost are cousins!

6. Now focus on the umbilical center of your body. Sense any connection you may notice from it to the periphery of your

body-being. Notice center and periphery: your body as a cell.

7. Now we'll focus on any sense of connection between your navel center and your limbs. In this pattern, all the limbs have equal importance, like those of a starfish. We'll focus on all six limbs: your two arms, two legs, your head, and your tail as they each radiate from your navel center.

8. Beginning with awareness at your navel, sense along the line from it to the fingertips of your right hand. Now imagine you are breathing, or imagine your breath traveling, along this line. Inhale from your navel center out through the right hand's fingertips and exhale along this line back to your navel center. Sense any connectivity along this line. Is there any disconnection, any area that seems fuzzy or unclear, or a place where the breath (or image of the breath) seems to stop or has difficulty?

9. We'll explore each limb in the same manner. Bring your awareness to your navel and sense along the line from it to your head. Now imagine you are breathing, or imagine your breath traveling, along this line. Inhale from your navel center out through your head and exhale along this line back to your navel center. Sense any connectivity along this line. Is there any disconnection, any area that seems fuzzy or unclear, or a place where the breath (or image of the breath) seems to stop or has difficulty?

10. Now bring your awareness to your navel, and sense along the line from it to the fingertips of your left hand. Now imagine you are breathing, or imagine your breath traveling, along this line. Inhale from your navel center out through the left hand's fingertips, and exhale along this line back to your navel center. Sense any connectivity along this line. Is there any disconnection, any area that seems fuzzy or unclear,

or a place where the breath (or image of the breath) seems to stop or has difficulty?

11. Next bring your awareness to your navel along the line from it to the toes of your left foot. Now imagine you are breathing, or imagine your breath traveling, along this line. Inhale from your navel center out through the toes of the left foot, and exhale along this line back to your navel center. Sense any connectivity along this line. Is there any disconnection, any area that seems fuzzy or unclear, or a place where the breath (or image of the breath) seems to stop or has difficulty?

12. Now bring your awareness to your navel along the line from it to the fingertips of your coccyx. Now imagine you are breathing, or imagine your breath traveling, along this line. Inhale from your navel center out through the coccyx, and exhale along this line back to your navel center. Sense any connectivity along this line. Is there any disconnection, any area that seems fuzzy or unclear, or a place where the breath (or image of the breath) seems to stop or has difficulty?

13. Last, bring awareness to your navel along the line from it to the toes of your right foot. Now imagine you are breathing, or imagine your breath traveling, along this line. Inhale from your navel center out through the toes of the right foot, and exhale along this line back to your navel center. Sense any connectivity along this line. Is there any disconnection, any area that seems fuzzy or unclear, or a place where the breath (or image of the breath) seems to stop or has difficulty?

What did you discover? Were there any areas of disconnect or confusion of throughline? Can you think of any reason for this? What is your movement and coordination like along this line? If this exploration was of interest to you, consider exploring combinations of the limbs that replicate movement patterns you know or would like to improve. For instance, consider your seated posture. What do you do to achieve it and what might help improve it?

VERTEBRATE PATTERNS

The next four patterns are vertebrate patterns that can be seen in the performance of the practice of *yogasana* and *vinyasa*. It is not that there is necessarily a one-to-one correspondence throughout all the poses, yet there are some pretty clear matches between *yogasana* and *vinyasa* and pre-vertebrate and vertebrate patterns. The organization and movement qualities of the pre-vertebrate patterns underlie and thus support the vertebrate patterns. In fact one of the premises of this work, as it is developmental, is that when there is an issue presenting in a pattern one may look to the pattern or patterns that precede it for clues as to what might be awry. These patterns align well with my organization by midline category as they all organize around the body's midline.

For these patterns, five basic actions of yielding, pushing, reaching, grasping, and pulling, which we'll explore further in the next chapter, initiate the movement and affect the way the pattern is sequenced through the body. If you wish to explore these patterns further, you may want to spend time trying out the five actions in your various limbs (including the head and tail) to see how your body best organizes for their use.

The vertebrate patterns came into importance when creatures came out of the water to negotiate survival on land. In a similar way, when we are born most of us are pushed out headward from a fluid matrix into a world of gravity and space. Our skeletal system provides the scaffolding around which we organize our movement both away and toward. We gradually build strength as we navigate the use of our head, spine, torso, and limbs. Then with the spinal midline as the point of orientation, we gain ability and then skill in the various coordinated uses of the four limbs, developing increasingly nuanced and complex movement phrases.

Spinal patterns sequence through the vertebrae and organize pathways along the core. These are seen in creatures without limbs such as fish and snakes. Homologous patterns of the limbs differentiate movement between the upper and lower body and can be seen in amphibians like frogs. Homolateral patterns differentiate movement on the right and left sides of the body and are seen in reptiles like lizards. And contralateral patterns establish diagonal connections across the midline from the upper quadrant to its lower opposite. These patterns are seen in mammals.

Spinal

The spinal pattern is characterized by a strong central support. Many yoga poses utilize the spinal pattern as a baseline. This pattern is very important in all meditative poses and in proper *pranayama* practice. We as humans can both push from our head and tail and reach from our head and tail. The push patterns take us into an experience of compression while the reach patterns into elongation. Therefore the push patterns can be seen as the precursors for strength, with the reach patterns precursors for lightness and articulation in space.

Homologous

Homologous patterns organize the whole-body using flexion and extension in the sagittal plane.

This is a symmetrical pattern in that both arms and both legs move simultaneously and mirror each other. The midline is an important center of this symmetry. This pattern establishes lateral stability throughout the body. It differentiates the upper from the lower.

Homolateral

The homolateral pattern differentiates the two sides, right and left, of the body with the vertical axis as the dividing line. When in play, it organizes the whole body to enable side–side asymmetrical weight shift. Along with this we may see lateral flexion of the torso as well as adduction and abduction.

Contralateral

The contralateral pattern differentiates the four quadrants of the body: the right upper torso and limb, the left upper torso and limb, the right lower torso and limb, and the left lower torso and limb. As a whole-body pattern, it establishes the diagonal connections between upper and lower limbs: right upper with left lower, and left upper with right lower. Mammals rely on this pattern to lift each foot independently. Twists and spiraling movements utilize this pattern.

Humans pass through all these patterns as they develop to bipedal standing and locomotion. Even when moving on two feet, the organization and sequencing of the limbs determine the pattern used:

- homologous as in jumping
- homolateral as in hopping on one foot
- contralateral as in leaping from one foot to the other.

SOMATIC PRACTICE: Organization around the midline

1. Stand and locate in your body the vertical dimension from the top of your head to your pelvic floor or tail. Notice how you maintain this position. Are you pushing, or reaching in some way at either end of your body, or with some part or parts of your body? Are you releasing into gravity and/or into space? As you sense this vertical axis, notice which parts of your body run along its line, i.e., which parts are organized near and around it.

2. Allow yourself to tilt off the vertical dimension and return to it. Without taking a step, begin to move your arms and spine so you go farther out into the space around you and return back to this central shaft. Notice how the vertical is a base from which you can move away and to which you can return.

3. Now bring your attention to the front of your body from about the middle of your body forward. Feel this area and notice your response to it. Initiate movement from the front body. Move forward from it. Move backward from it. What does this feel like and remind you of? What is your sense of the value or usefulness of this part of your body? See if you can initiate any movement from this part only. What else do you notice there?

4. Now pay attention to the back part of your body from the middle to the back. Notice what this aspect of your body feels like. Initiate movement from the back body. Move backward from it. Move forward from it. What does this feel like and remind you of? What is your sense of the value or usefulness of this part of your body? See if you can initiate any movement from this part only. What else do you notice there?

5. Now focus on the middle of your body, as in the central tissues sandwiched between front and back. Move about and notice the import of this layer of your body. Notice/imagine/visualize/feel a central line or

channel within. You may at first wish to examine it as an energetic pathway: a channel for energy. We can call this, generally speaking, the Shushumna Nadi. You know it as the primary *nadi* of the three main *nadis* (channels of energy) in the body. As the central channel, Shushumna Nadi runs straight up the center of the body, and connects each of the chakras like jewels on a strand. On the physical level, an early manifestation of the midline is the notochord. It extends from the head to the tail. The midline is necessary for orientation in space and gravity and is the basis for organized movement.

6. Still standing, allow your body to fold forward in a way that is comfortable to you. Notice your sense of right–left symmetry, and your balance as your head moves off vertical as you descend. What actions are you using to perform this movement? What else do you notice? Return to standing.

7. Next allow your body to go into a back bend that is comfortable for you. This may only be to look upward with your head supported by your hands clasped behind it. Notice again your ability to balance as you move, your weight shifting as you do so, and your sense of symmetry. What else occurs to you? Return to standing.

8. Next bend to one side; you may choose to raise one or both arms overhead, place them on your hips, or simply let them dangle. Notice again your sense of balance as you move. What happens to your weight and to the lower end of your spine? What do you wish to happen? Repeat this on the opposite side. Notice any difference?

9. Now rotate your head and upper body comfortably to the right. Reach the arms out a bit or place the hands on the hips as you like. Notice the midline as you revolve. Do parts of your body come off midline as you turn? If so, why do they do so? How is your weight distributed? How is your balance? Could you walk forward with this configuration of your body? What adjustments might you make to do so?

The assorted *yogasana* and *vinyasa* movements call upon various organizations of these basic patterns. Explore the poses and *vinyasas* you practice regularly with these four patterns of spinal, homologous, homolateral, and contralateral in mind. Discern which patterns you employ to accomplish each yoga posture. If you can, observe others in their practice. What patterns do you see in what the pose they perform demands? What do you see underlying? If the posture or movement looks awry or in some way off or unsupported, what might be missing? Which pattern or patterns could give more integrity to the performance of the pose or movement? What reason might there be to choose one pattern over another?

Looking at body organization is an important aspect of yoga therapy in that it can address issues of dysfunctional patterning and correct movement problems that lead to misalignment, compensatory body use, subsequent pain, and further dysfunction. Looking in particular at specific action patterning, or at whole-body use, can give insight into distinct weaknesses, areas of congestion, or movement gaps in development, all of which may play a part in an individual's ability to find ease and comfort in their own movement signature. In the next chapter we'll look at the character of the movement more closely and its potential to give even more refined ability to design yoga-based movement practices that target the tissues and patterns of use in need or remedy.

CHAPTER 6

Embodying Movement Quality

What gives us motivation to move? What is the inner urging that takes us off our seat into action in space? In yoga philosophy we have the notions of *raga* and *dvesha*, attraction and aversion. We want and we avoid. When I first learned these terms, it brought to mind a film I'd seen of a microscopic creature under a microscope streaming in a favorable direction while withdrawing from a noxious stimulant in its environment. As I recall there was an easy gentleness to the friendly space and what looked like a hurried contraction away from the unfriendly one.

The term movement quality may evoke the image of virtuosity in performance—whether in an athlete, musician, or surgeon. Efficient movement is the effect of combining optimal differentiation, support, and organization in producing movement. Woven into expert movement skill is a more fine-tuned use of the idea of the quality of the movement. It is to consider the movement's dynamics by looking at the changeable features of a movement, the "how" of its execution as it reveals the inner attitude of the mover. What is the mover's approach to what they are doing? What is the mark of their inner world on their actions? And what does the movement reveal about them? In this chapter we'll explore two taxonomies of the expressive aspects of movement dynamics, or quality of movement, that can be

applied as useful features of effecting movement efficiency in yoga therapy.

In our early life, as our faculties are developing, we move toward and away in a similar fashion. We, like other creatures, have a series of reflexes that arise, which organize our body to do things automatically like flex, extend, grasp, and suck. These responses integrate into a more complex matrix of options in our developing movement repertoire. The success of this integration is based on many things. For instance, is our environment hostile or friendly? Is our drive for exploration met with satisfaction or thwarted with frustration and disappointment? When our needs are expressed, are they met? Because movement is the medium of our early life, it is where and how we first meet our world. The arc of the expression of our desires—to go toward or away—in movement will begin to be laid down as a pattern of interaction that will continue to shape our way of relating in the world. In later life these strategies are apparent in our movement dynamics, in the way we inhabit our body and expend our energy, and in our ability to manage our nervous system and our mind and emotions. All this patterning begins in these early arcs of interaction, and whether we can succeed in being met well enough by our environs.

THE FIVE BASIC ACTIONS OF THE SATISFACTION CYCLE

The satisfaction cycle, as taught by Bonnie Bainbridge Cohen, identifies five specific basic neurological actions or types of movement (Schwartz, 2018). The actions can be seen as progressing from one to the next, in a sequence that leads to getting what one wants, hence satisfaction results.

I consider it a taxonomy in that all movement can be described as a simple or complex performance of its five actions. The actions are also considered developmental, in that each is thought to underlie and support the next in a sequential chain of doing. The actions in the cycle are yield, push, reach, grasp, and pull. Acceptance of success could result in a yield, which may begin a new cycle. The idea here is that each movement you do is going to involve these five actions in a dizzying array of possible combinations. And yet, with careful observation, an individual's characteristic use of them may issue forth as a signature of their way of moving in the world and strategies for coping with not only the environment of gravity and space, but the people and things in it.

If I'm not able to settle myself well enough to fall asleep, then I may be able to work with yielding as a somatic practice. Or, if I'm not able to stand up for myself in conflict or have the courage to speak, I may work with pushing as an abstraction, not as a thought, but as a movement engendering a bodily felt sense.

Looking at movement through the lens of my orientation to and habitual use of the five basic actions can give me insight into what I used early on to solve the challenges in my early life before I could talk in words and use top-down coaching. My movement life is how I'm organized to meet my world. So working with this can help me repattern this in my adult here and now. We'll briefly explore each action below. If you respond to working with one or more of these actions, please take the time, now or later, to investigate what your embodied responses are about for you.

Yield

As a word, yield may evoke several associations. For me, stopping to let other drivers go by is what at first comes to mind. Another may be of oppression, being forced to give up something in defeat. What the word indicates somatically here is rooted in surrender but in a cooperative way—more in the nature of a receptive exchange than a forced march. My experience of yielding is giving up control while gaining support. Yielding can be into gravity, as when you take a step with a bent leg to leap upward, or it can be into space, like when you first see someone you love and move toward them to embrace. It's a pleasure to go into both of these willingly, and there is a return on investment. Cohen makes the point of distinguishing this from collapse, which in my experience does not have a sense of gradated release and attentiveness but is more of a dropping of everything when one's efforts can no longer be maintained.

Push

A more readily recognized action, to push is to exert force to move away or to move something else away. It has the power to separate and takes effort. Physically pushing uses muscles and organizes the body around a center for greater control of force. It has an enlivening and engaging effect.

Reach

In reaching we attend to what is beyond us and move out into space. As we do so, our ability to support going beyond ourselves comes into play. Curiosity and connection, satisfaction and investigation all come into range as our reach mobilizes us into engagement with our world.

Grasp

In common parlance we may be more likely to refer to grasping something intellectually, like a concept we understand, rather than to physically grab hold. In movement, a grasp happens when some part of the mover's body encloses around an object. The object may be an immovable one that we might draw our body toward, or an object that we draw to us, or hold at the original length. It may, as in the case of a yoga pose, be a different part of our own body, or even a space within it. *Mula bandha* (the root lock), in which we grasp

with the pelvic floor, is not so much grasping an object as performing a grasping motion in space within the body.

Pull

To pull is to lessen the distance between ourselves and something else. We pull a movable object closer or, if it's fixed in place, we pull our body closer to it. Pulling completes the action sequence of the satisfaction cycle, with the possibility of yielding again to receive what it is we have been after in the first place.

SOMATIC PRACTICE: The five basic actions

1. Begin lying on the floor in the way you are most comfortable. Feel the body's weight and allow each body area to yield into the floor beneath you. Begin with your head. Notice its weight and the surface of the floor where your head makes contact. Allow the weight of the head to sink into the floor, as when you step into soft sand. Continue to the neck, even though it is suspended off the floor, allow its weight to fall into the field of gravity, like a suspension bridge. Continue through the torso, allowing the weight to yield as best you can. Include your arms, allowing gravity to hold them. Travel into the lower back and pelvic area, releasing your weight. Sense it and allow it to release into gravity. Take your time. Then travel through your legs and feet, letting them yield as well. Allow the earth to fully hold your body.

2. Next, bring your attention to the space you occupy. Feel the volume of your body and notice the space it takes up. Then notice the space just outside of your body, a few inches to a foot around you. Breathe and relax and feel your attention inhabit this space around you. If you like you can continue to expand your attention further out into the space that surrounds you. Feel that you are in the space, that the space is inviting, and you are aware of it.

3. Notice if there is any particular place or area of the space around that has special interest for you. Or maybe there is something or someone in the space that catches your interest. Allow yourself to turn to look or turn in response to your curiosity and interest in that location. What do you notice? Is this in any way familiar to you?

4. When you're ready, focus on a body area in which you feel you have good contact with the earth through the surface you are on, such as the floor or your mat. Let that feeling of contact turn into a push with that part. This may be a part of your body you are not used to pushing with, like the center of your back, the side of your head, or your calf. As if you are new to the world, if you can, allow yourself to notice what it feels like for you to push with this body part. Try a different part as well. See what you notice.

5. When you are ready, change your position so you can arrange your body in a more

familiar way so that you can push with your hands, feet, forearms, or shins. Push in ways you enjoy or find interesting. Notice your response to pushing in this way. Do you want to add any sound? Does a yoga pose emerge? Is there a rhythm to it? How do you find pushing? Tiring? Enlivening? When you are happy enough with pushing, allow your body to relax again. Pause your activity and sense. What do you notice? Is there any emotion? And recollection of a time when you used pushing? What associations, memories, and feelings arise for you just now?

6. Next choose an object that appeals to you and is near enough that you could eventually touch and grasp. If you need, pause in the exploration to set up something within your reach.

7. One caveat about reaching is that it tends to go better when you have yielding and pushing as resources underlying this action of moving away from self into untested space. Here you can explore that postulate by reaching without reconnection to the earth and using pushing in coordination.

That is, try an unsupported reach. Then go back and feel again your contact to the earth, feel the support and organization pushing off gives you, and then reach for the object. Or just begin with this if you prefer.

8. Once you have reached your object, slow down to slow motion if you can. Observe the moment when you close your hand or body around the object you've desired. What does that feel like in your body? What memories, if any, come to mind? Is there any emotion? What do you notice?

9. Now pull the object toward you, or, if it is stationary, pull yourself to it. Once you've brought the object close, notice again what happens in your experience. Do you experience the satisfaction of getting what you've wanted? Notice any other feelings that arise. For instance, is there sadness, fear, frustration, or confusion. Take time to notice your response to each of these actions. Feel free to go back through them, focusing on each one as they are of interest to you.

Because "everything is everything," as the saying goes, we can see that our movement not only portrays mechanical efficiency but is also expressive of inner attitude. As we work to repattern ineffective movement and body use we open the door to our feeling life and how movement serves as a means of functioning. Our movement patterns reflect our decisions and strategies for engaging in our world.

In exploring these five basic actions in our training programs, at times we'll collect reflections on their experience in the form of very short verbal expressions. Here are some from our students.

Verbal responses to embodying: Yield

Relaxed and aware	Resting in contact	Being versus doing
Letting go of restrictions	Easy breathing	Nice
Safe and secure	Attachment	Homey
Not stressed out	Trusting	Being held
Belonging	Cared for	Welcoming
Foundation	Grounding	Enjoined with
Supported	Registering safety	Melting

Verbal responses to embodying: Push

Strength	Powerful	Activating
Asserting myself	Willfulness	Muscles working
Densify	Internal support	Confidence
Being substantial	Sense of self	Ability to separate
Weight	Standing up for myself	Wrestling
Saying I am here	"No." "Not you—me."	Weight training
Doing squats	Gravitas	For boundaries

Verbal responses to embodying: Reach

Wanting something	Excitement	Following curiosity
Being outward focused	Saying yes!	Exposure
Following passion	Going out	Aiming
Risking engagement	Risking rejection	Mobilizing
Expressing needs	Just outside comfort zone	Going for it
Having goals you're not sure you can get	The unknown	

Verbal responses to embodying: Grasp

Getting it	A good grip	Claiming ownership
Manifesting desire	Achievement	Holding it
Learning	Surrounding	Control of something
Having in hand	Ownership	Command

Verbal responses to embodying: Pull

Assimilating	Taking it home	Taking in from external
Taking the win	Resting in what I have	Meeting
Power to bring toward	Accomplishment	Bringing together/closer

Even though our focus is on movement efficiency, the expressive aspect of movement quality or its dynamics is an inseparable aspect of movement life. Movement is implicitly expressive. The space we use has a character to it. Up is up and down is down. And the dynamics implicit in our every movement do too. These five actions are developmental but not in a linear way. They arise like waves on the shoreline, with one withdrawing while another becomes more pronounced; they overlap, having an ebb and flow.

If we have a good enough early movement life, with enough safe exploration in a friendly enough environment, we'll have a good basis for each aspect of the satisfaction cycle to be enacted in our development. If our early ability to move and explore is disrupted or inhibited in some way, we may notice, as we examine our embodied experience of these actions, something awry.

In yoga therapy we often begin on the physical level with the physical sheath, because that is where aches and pains become noticeable. As we work to understand what patterns underly the use of our bodies, we may uncover feeling sensation, interoceptive data, that recounts for us some displaced satisfaction in our efforts to move, live, and thrive. These may manifest as movement inhibition, lack of physically aligned support, confusion of initiation, ineffective use of dynamics, and lack of functional application of these five actions, among other things. We can observe movement, make suggestions for reorganization, and train for functional efficiency. In doing so, it's wise to also acknowledge that a host of feelings, of nonverbal memories, of interrupted or thwarted movement attempts in early life, may as well have a causal role to play.

OBSERVATION OF THE FIVE BASIC ACTION ANALYSIS OF MOVEMENT SKILL: THE CASE OF MARCUS

Marcus, a 17-year-old male with he/his pronouns, and a varsity basketball player, was a patient of a physical therapy practice that also offers athletic training. Marcus had repeated problems with shin splints and knee pain. The trainer had been working with his lay-ups and jump shots and was working on his stride and propulsion going into the lay-ups when I joined them. I noticed that Marcus was efficient in his organization and had accuracy in his aim, but that after he shot the ball it was as if he let go of all that clarity in space and attention to the space around him and dropped to the ground in almost a state of collapsed relief. This was his recuperation, for certain, which made sense, but he was landing hard on his whole foot without awareness of how he landed.

We worked with foot-strike, exploring landing by rolling through the foot rather than landing as one flat surface, but, when it was time to put that into practice, he became rigid in his approach to using his legs, adding more tension in an effort to get it right. This was noticeably worse. We then did a relaxation practice that verbally directed Marcus through the sensation of yielding systematically through each body area. He was then asked to notice how he felt afterwards. We discussed being aware of releasing into the floor or ground without collapsing while doing so, paying attention without controlling. He immediately associated this feeling with shooting the ball. Even though this was a push of an object through space at a very specific target, he felt he also needed to release into the space as he shot, or he would create too much tension and miss the basket.

We then took this sensation of releasing with attention into very small jumps and landings, barely getting off the floor. I coached his landings, asking him to release with attention, which were his words. I eventually asked if he noticed whether this was better on his knees or worse, and to verbalize how it felt so he could find this experience again in the future.

I gave him these little "soft jumps," as we called them, for homework until our next session. When he came back at the end of the week he proudly demonstrated his lay-up with a fully functional landing of yielding into the floor with his weight traveling through the bones, not being stopped by tension, rolling toe–ball–heel into the floor. We continued to work on his spatial awareness of his body's weight as he tried different versions of shooting and landing, to further apply and integrate the pattern, and bring even more awareness of alignment into the mix. His PT/trainer adeptly guided him in ways to not overtrain and, as far as I know, he has not had any further problems with his shins and knees.

With Marcus we didn't enter into the yielding as a pattern for deeper exploration of self and life strategy, but it may come up for him later. It is hard to know whether a physical learning will translate into a metaphorical or even metaphysical one, or whether it needs to do so for someone to benefit.

Through the five basic actions we have seen how the effectiveness of one developmental movement can rely upon a prior one in efficient movement patterning. Working with these five actions can be a way to learn more about your early movement life and environment. Movement efficiency can be improved by looking at the use of these actions when pain or dysfunction happens. It's important to recognize movement as not only a mechanical process but also as an expression of the mover's felt experience. Features of how movement is performed reveal early decisions based on felt responses to the degree of satisfaction and success in movement into one's world in early life.

Observation of movement patterning can be layered into related psychological, trauma, and developmental histories with resonant patterning prevailing across models. Patterns of inefficiency and impediment can be worked with directly through movement. One might explore them through *asana* and *vinyasa*, relaxation and breathing, mindfulness in actions and in inter-actions, or in simply examining the effectiveness of daily actions and the state of being one is in while performing them. In the next section below we'll go more deeply into the expression of inner attitudes as they are expressed in the dynamics of movement.

LABAN MOVEMENT ANALYSIS IN REFINING MOVEMENT QUALITY AND DEVELOPING SKILL

Over the years, Rudolph Laban's system of move-ment analysis has been encapsulated in a method called Laban Movement Analysis. It has four main areas: body, space, shape, and effort, effort being synonymous with movement quality. Here, as above, movement quality is seen as the expres-sion of inner attitudes or states of being, such as being peaceful or rushed, hostile, frightened, or calm, as these feeling states become visible in physical posture and movement dynamics. These areas of movement have had diverse applications in psychology, yoga and movement therapy, health, dance, theater, art, industry, business management, and more. The four main catego-ries interrelate and are integral in that our body: (1) exists in space, (2) has form or shape and when moving, (3) moves with some dynamism, even if at times this is minimal.

Body

Body refers to body part awareness and use dur-ing movement, including initiation, sequencing, relation of body parts in action and in spatial configuration, "kinetic chains" or connectivity of action, and alignment in relation to main body areas in stillness and in movement as reflected in efficient functioning.

Shape

Shape refers to the sculptural forms the body takes in its spatial environment. (The subcategories of these are called modes of shape change: shape flow, directional, and shaping.) We solve move-ment situations by possessing an attitude, mostly unconscious or even reflexive, toward shape, i.e., we shape our bodies automatically according to our situation. For example, most of us will mold our chest and arm around the tiny form of the newborn we are invited to hold.

Space

Space refers to the space in and around the body and the spatial forms created through movement. Laban relates the body's sculptural form and its part's movement pathways to the Platonic Solids, such as the cube, the tetrahedron, and the 20-sided icosahedrons, and others to the space we may move into and travel through in our kinesphere. He created space "scales" and "chords," similar in a sense to musical "scales" and "chords," which were the basis of his movement "choirs," and called this study "space harmony."

Effort

Effort (*Antrieb* in German) refers to movement quality and dynamics, or the expressive aspect of movement. Through effort, or a movement's dynamic quality, feeling, emotion, subtext, and in part psychological content are communicated. It's expressive of the mover's drive or inner impulse to act.

THE FIGHTING–INDULGING CONTINUUM OF LABAN'S EFFORT

Movement is a psychophysical phenomenon. It involves the whole person. The language of our body *is* movement, and it often speaks much louder than words. An individual's feeling state, or, as Laban called it, their inner attitude, becomes observable through the quality of their movement. Laban termed inner attitudes as revealed in movement "effort."

To articulate movement quality, which I'll now refer to as effort, Laban identified the four motion factors of weight or force, space, time, and flow. He organized the notable attributes of these factors on a continuum from indulging in them to fighting against or resisting them. Laban believed that a mover adopts a fighting or indulging attitude toward each motion factor. So the motion factors exist on a continuum of opposites. For instance, if I have an indulgent attitude toward time, I will move slowly with no haste. If I have a fighting attitude, I will hurriedly run against time.

Weight refers to the amount of exertion. It is felt in one's own body and observed in others, existing on a continuum of strong to light. A fighting attitude is expressed as *strong* weight characterized by forcefulness and exertion. An indulging attitude is expressed as *light* weight, involving delicacy, softness, and gentleness. There is also the possibility of a neutral amount of weight or force (these terms of weight and force can be used interchangeably). In this case, the force used for an action is neither strong nor light and is simply not noted.

Space is the effort that orients movement. It's felt in one's own bodily awareness and observed externally in others on a continuum of direct, as in aiming linearly, to indirect, using curving, scattering, and multidirectional changes and attention.

Time is felt in one's own body and observed in others on a continuum of quick (also called sudden) to slow (also called sustained).

And *flow* is the effort exerted to control movement. It's felt in one's own bodily experience and observed externally in others on a continuum of bound to free. In bound flow, motion can be stopped or is restrained at any moment. In free flow, action is relaxed and fluid and is difficult to stop suddenly.

These various levels of differentiation leave us with the resulting attributes, called the effort elements, of strong to light, direct to indirect, fast to slow, and bound to free. Placing the elements on the continuum of each motion factor gives insight into the mover's inner attitude about the use of each one. Please be reminded that inner attitudes are mostly unconscious until they are made conscious.

The effort elements on the continuum of Laban's motion factors

Motion factor	Effort elements		
Force	Strong	(Neutral)	Light
Space	Direct	(Neutral)	Indirect
Time	Quick/Sudden	(Neutral)	Slow/Sustained
Flow	Bound	(Neutral)	Free

Any movement you do can be tracked on some part of the continuum for each motion factor. Say your cat knocks your teacup from the table where you're sitting. You see this out of the corner of your eye and move to catch the cup before it shatters on the floor. It's likely you moved quickly and directly to catch the cup. Your movement was probably stronger than it was lighter because if you are like most people, there is an affinity between moving quickly and directly and strength. And your flow may have begun as free, but ended up more bound as you would need to control the cup, catching it without breaking it in your hand.

So the profile for this action of teacup catching may have been something like:

Motion factor	Effort elements
Weight	*Strong*
Space	*Direct*
Time	*Quick*
Flow	*Bound*

As you consider this, it's likely to occur to you that our bodies evoke an ocean of ever-changing movement dynamics, with overlapping phrases, accelerations and decelerations, and all manner of change between these elements as we move throughout our day. Laban separated these elements out to differentiate them. Thus we can analyze the movement with great specificity. In reality they appear in our movement merged together. Laban devised terminology and a notation system that allowed for combinations of the effort elements to be observed and recorded. A finer point on phrasing of movement dynamics being general or specific can be made; suffice it to say that his method could be used to capture very fine details of movement as it is articulated in a body or bodies, or general, wide-angled themes or motifs as the purpose of the capture required.

So, taking for a moment the eight effort elements, on the continuum of each one's motion factor of weight, space, time, and flow, we can consider the efficient use of each one. The idea here in observing movement, is whether the mover is using these motion factors well enough, or even optimally, as in the case of high-level skill such as in athletic or artistic performance. And if not, why not? What could be the cause? The cause may or may not be apparent at the moment of observation, but the practice of observing gives us the information we need to assess efficiency through this lens of movement quality.

Let's return to the teacup catch as the movement we're observing. In terms of the timing, did the mover respond in time? Was the movement too fast or too slow? In this situation, if the mover was, for instance, way too slow, it begs the question of why was that so? We wonder, when the teacup shatters, what was the issue? Was the movement too strong, too light, or was it just right? In terms of space, was the mover able to get their hand in place, organizing their attention, and then their body, to move it there directly, or did they miss and by how much space? And with flow between bound and free, was the movement too rigid or too free flowing, i.e., was the movement done within the range of good control? If not, in any one or more of these we have something awry that is worth investigating.

We make these observations instinctually all the time as part of our everyday read on the people in our field of experience. We go to the shop and notice someone's movement seems a bit odd. We check them out to see if they're alright or if they present any danger. This is all registering below our conscious mind. Knowing the motion factors and their elements gives us a way to articulate what we are in fact seeing. What exactly is off? In yoga therapy, with this awareness of movement elements, we can assess to a very fine level if need be, and work to uncover the causal factors in the movement repertoire of our clients.

SOMATIC PRACTICE: Motion factor

In this exploration we'll take the motion factors one by one and slide from one polar element to its opposite along its continuum. Take your time with this and see if you can notice what other elements come along as you attempt to embody just one of them. Also, you're likely to find that the fighting elements are tiring! So please do as little or as much movement as you like within your comfortable capacity. Have fun with it! To get the full gestalt, if possible stand and move with your whole body. If that isn't right for you just now, please note that you can do this work with one limb, or even one finger!

1. Beginning with weight effort, feel the strength of your body—whatever that means to you. Now move in a way that uses strong effort. Do the strongest movements you can within your capacity. Make sounds if you like, breathe! Interact with objects. Feel the power! Now allow this to diminish gradually until you are moving with a more or less neutral attitude toward weight.

2. Notice what other elements supported your expression of strength. What does this effort element of strength feel like to you? Is it familiar and if so in what ways? What does it remind you of? How does it serve you in your life just now? Could you use more or less of it in your movement, your body, your life?

3. Now move from strength into lightness at the other end of the weight effort continuum. Feel lightness in your body—whatever that means to you. Now move in a way that uses light effort. Do the lightest movements you can. Make sounds if you like, breathe! Interact with objects if you like. Now allow this to diminish gradually until you are moving with a more or less neutral attitude toward weight.

4. Notice what other elements supported your expression of lightness. Is there a preferred place in space in which you tend to move when you move with lightness? What does this effort element of lightness feel like to you? Is it familiar and if so in what ways? What does it remind you of? How does it serve you in your life just now? Could you use more or less of it in your movement, your body, your life?

5. Now focus on space effort, which is a continuum of direct use of space to indirect all-around awareness of and investment in space. Begin with direct movement. Move directly in space. Use your limbs, your whole body, several parts together as you like. Make sounds if you like, breathe! Interact with objects as you wish. Now allow this to diminish gradually until you are moving with a more or less neutral attitude toward space.

6. Notice what other elements supported your expression of directness. Is there a preferred place in space in which you tend to move when you move with directness? What does this effort element of directness feel like to you? Is it familiar and if so in what ways? What does it remind you of? How does it serve you in your life just now? Could you use more or less of it in your movement, your body, your life?

7. Now transition from direct movement to indirect movement on the space effort continuum. Move indirectly in space. Use your limbs, your whole body, and several parts together to move indirectly in space. Make sounds if you like, breathe! Interact with objects as you wish. Now allow this to diminish gradually until you are moving with a more or less neutral attitude toward space.

8. Notice what other elements supported your expression of indirectness. Are there preferred places in space in which you tend to move when you move with indirectness? What does this effort element of indirectness feel like to you? Is it familiar and if so in what ways? What does it remind you of? How does it serve you in your life just now? Could you use more or less of it in your movement, your body, your life?

9. Now we'll move on to the motion factor of time, beginning with quickness. Feel the preparation for quick movement in your body. Now move in a way that uses quickness. Do the fastest movements you can within your capacity. Make sounds if you like, breathe! Interact with objects. Feel the speed! Now allow this to diminish gradually until you are moving with a more or less neutral attitude toward time.

10. Notice what other elements supported your expression of quickness. What does this effort element of quickness feel like to you? Is it familiar and if so in what ways? What does it remind you of? How does it serve you in your life just now? Could you use more or less of it in your movement, your body, your life?

11. Now we'll move on to the opposite element of motion factor of time, slowness, or sustained movement. Feel the preparation for slow movement in your body. Now move slowly. Do the slowest movements you can. Make sounds if you like, breathe! Interact with objects. Feel the sustained quality of slow movement. Now allow this to diminish gradually until you are moving with a more or less neutral attitude toward time.

12. Notice what other elements supported your expression of slowness. What does this effort element of slowness feel like to you? Is it familiar and if so in what ways? What does it remind you of? How does it serve you in your life just now? Could you use more or less of it in your movement, your body, your life?

13. Turning attention to the motion factor of flow, we'll explore the effort element of bound flow. Feel the binding of flow in your body—whatever that means to you. Now move in a way that uses bound flow; this is movement that you could stop at any moment. Do the most bound movements you can within your capacity. Make sounds if you like, breathe! Interact with objects. Feel the control! Now allow this to diminish gradually until you are moving with a more or less neutral attitude toward flow.

14. Notice what other elements supported your expression of bound flow. What does this effort element of bound flow feel like to you? Is it familiar and if so in what ways? What does it remind you of? How does it serve you in your life just now? Could you use more or less of it in your movement, your body, your life?

15. At the opposite end of the motion factor continuum of flow, we'll explore the effort element of free flow. Feel free flow in your body—whatever that means to you. Now move in a way that uses free flow. Do the most freely flowing movements you can. Make sounds if you like, breathe! Interact with objects. Feel the freedom! Now allow this to diminish gradually until you are moving with a more or less neutral attitude toward flow.

16. Notice what other elements supported your expression of free flow. What does this effort element of free flow feel like to you? Is it familiar and if so in what ways? What does it remind you of? How does it serve you in your life just now? Could you use more or less of it in your movement, your body, your life?

17. When you are finished moving and ready to reflect, take each element one at a time and ask yourself: What sort of yoga therapy client would benefit from this effort element of: strength, lightness, directness, indirectness, quickness, slowness, binding control, or freedom of flow, for what challenge, and in what context?

THE EIGHT BASIC EFFORT ACTIONS OR DRIVES

We've just explored the individual effort elements on the continuum of the four motion factors of weight, space, time, and flow. As noted above, our movement exhibits these motion factors to greater or lesser degrees of intensity in varying rhythms and combinations in *all* our movements.

As we saw above, tracking a single element gives specific information regarding the use of that element. We can also observe the elements in combination, which is mostly what we see in movement. For various reasons, Laban eliminated flow as a defining feature of what he called the Eight Basic Effort Actions, so they result from all the possible combinations of weight, space, and time. Combining the elements gives a sort of shorthand for identifying movement qualities.

Also, the level of intensity of feeling can be observed in the number of effort elements seen. Without going too far into this, suffice it to say that we can make note of intensity. When three effort elements of an effort action are present, we are fully invested in the feeling of the movement; it takes us over, so to speak; we are "totally in" the feeling of it. Laban called this a drive. When only two effort elements predominate in a movement, we have dialed back our involvement a tad. The movement feels and reads as less intense. Laban called these states. They are seen more in the normal zone of daily activities.

SOMATIC PRACTICE: The Eight Basic Effort Actions

To arrive at the Eight Basic Effort Actions, which are combinations of the three effort elements of weight, space, and time, one simply combines one element from each motion factor. Try each combination below in movement and once you do, see what you would name the resultant action below.

1. Strong, direct, and quick:

   ....

2. Strong, direct, and slow:

   ....

3. Strong, indirect, and quick:

   ....

4. Strong, indirect, and slow:

   ....

5. Light, direct, and quick:

   ....

6. Light, direct, and slow:

   ....

7. Light, indirect, and quick:

   ....

8. Light, indirect, and slow:

   ....

Laban named the above combinations as follows: (1) punch, (2) press, (3) slash, (4) wring, (5) dab, (6) glide, (7) flick, and (8) float. Were your names for these combinations similar to Laban's?

Laban went on to discuss affinities between these movement qualities and space in the kinesphere. Learning these movements and locations by rote, while at first seeming the epitome of abstraction, can be an excellent way to embody them for the sake of observation and use in mediation of movement efficiency issues. For now, without going into that level of detail, we'll look at how movement dynamics can serve the yoga therapist in application.

If you were able to give the somatization above a full-bodied try, you can clearly see that movement not only expresses inner states but evokes them in us as well. The maxim "act your way to a feeling" in this case extends to the character or effort experience the movement engenders. Perhaps a person who is stuck and rigidly unable to change could be helped by exploring movement that is characterized by free flow with quick, light directional changes. To experience this in their body—would it not influence their mind and psyche as well? Or take someone confounded by despair and an inability to activate. Could they not benefit from movement that has directness and takes them from lightness to strength? Or any other manner of investigation and response within an individual struggling to find new avenues to *move* into new behavior. The physical is the metaphysical, our bodily experience feeds into our psyche and soul.

As far as movement skill and efficiency goes, working with the effort elements can bring a level of articulation to the therapeutic practices we give for specific purposes. The examples below are not prescriptive. Each effort combination would be tailored for each individual client, but they will give you an idea of the way this work could be utilized:

- For warming up arthritic joints: add the elements of indirectness and lightness into the joint capsule.
- For fascial congestion: use strong, direct, slow movement away from the line of pull of the main mover of the muscle group in question, and light, indirect, and slow movement in the opposite pathway.
- For overall high-tone muscle use: indirect, light, and quick movement with free flow as possible.
- For low muscle and autonomic tone: strong, bound, and quick movement, recuperating into light and free movement, done in an alternating, comfortable rhythm.
- For tissue experiencing pain and energetic stagnation: very light, slow, and indirect movement as tolerated in short bursts for not too much duration.

And on and on. Often remedial movement is given in terms of what body part moves where in space with the movement quality completely left to chance. Try doing your *asana* and *vinyasa* practice with attention to these effort features and see what ways you might alter the dynamics of your practice for greater benefit to you, your joints, muscles, organs, and other relevant tissues, as well as to your level of nuanced perception as you practice.

Developing and refining movement skill is an implicit part of every *asana* and *vinyasa* practice. It is also a huge part of helping clients with less than optimal body alignment and movement mechanics to improve their body use. Accurate application of effort qualities will not only act remedially as shown in the examples above but can also be the key to functional improvement in action patterning. The golf swing, the jump shot, the pirouette, and the dismount all require precise effort flow. Even picking up groceries or finding the best way to walk downstairs after a knee replacement can benefit from coaching of how to move, not just what goes where but *how*, for best results.

Section III

SOMATIC PRACTICE FOR SELF-INQUIRY AND REFLECTION

That which is worth taking up is the self-enquiry that reveals jnana; that which is worth enjoying is the grandeur of the Self; that which is worth renouncing is the ego-mind; that in which it is worth taking refuge, to eliminate sorrow completely, is one's own source, the Heart.

Ramana Maharshi (Godman, 2023)

INTRODUCTION: THE BODY AS MEDIUM FOR SELF-UNDERSTANDING AND PERSONAL TRANSFORMATION

Self-inquiry is an important aspect of yoga practice—although this may not be at first apparent from a Google search for yoga. In perhaps its purest form, *atman vichara,* literally meaning self-inquiry, is a process of discernment analyzing the source of our identity. Sri Ramana Maharshi and Nisargadatta Maharaj are two twentieth-century figures who brought this practice into more widespread contemporary use. Self-inquiry can also be something we use to discern which thoughts are useful to us and which are not. Within the context of yoga therapy, this practice of discernment can be deepened into in order to learn what is at the heart of an impediment to change in the direction we wish to go, rather than being stuck in a circular pattern of outworn habits that no longer serve our best selves.

Our experience of the body can be a rich resource for learning about these deeper habits of mind and emotion, as the body can hold the score and memory of our experiences at the cellular level. As Bonnie Bainbridge Cohen, the originator of Body-Mind Centering®, states, "Experience first occurs on the cellular level. The nervous system records the experience and organizes it into patterns" (Cohen, n.d., para. 1).

Embarking on the path of self-inquiry can take us out of our ordinary world of experience. In fact, this may just be a necessity in enacting the change we wish to achieve. To willingly and wittingly leave the safe and secure shoreline of known habits and ways of being, we must be ripe for the adventure. If we're lucky we'll be equipped with awareness and helped by allies and guides who know the way.

LEAVING THE SHORELINE TO RETURN RENEWED: THE HERO'S JOURNEY

The Hero's Journey is a set of concepts drawn from Carl G. Jung's depth psychology and the mythic studies of Joseph Campbell (Campbell, 1973). The claim is that it is an archetypal map of transformation with each person as the hero of their own story. This map is useful in that steps experienced over the course of meeting a life challenge, whether in the form of a relationship issue, an illness, or a global pandemic, are, with some variation, universal in nature. This story arc is not something made up as much as it is something discovered—a shared form of the internal experience of human nature.

The Hero's Journey describes the process of journeying and returning changed. In essence, it is the formula of passage of the soul through life, and on a lesser scale, through the trial of life events—not the least of which may be recovery from injury or illness. Joseph Campbell and his mentor Heinrich Zimmer, an authority on mythology, recognized that mythic stories, like those we piece together with our clients as they construct narratives that bring meaning to their struggle, are not mere whimsy. They are practical models of how human beings grow in the face of obstacles. Rudolph Ballentine's *Radical Healing* embraces this mythic journey by posing that illness and injury are opportunities, invitations even, to transform and evolve (Ballentine, 1999). In our work with clients this description of the process can guide us in tangible and reassuring ways as we assist our clients in opening to and examining deeper levels of being.

The Hero's Journey is articulated by Joseph Campbell in *The Hero with a Thousand Faces* (1973) in 17 stages. Others have used this soul journey in analyzing and designing plotlines from *The Wizard of Oz* to *Star Wars*. Christopher Vogler, in *The Writer's Journey* (Vogler, 2007, p. 6), outlines the sojourn in these 12 stages:

1. The Ordinary World
2. The Call to Adventure
3. The Refusal of the Call
4. Meeting the Mentor
5. Crossing the Threshold
6. Tests, Allies and Enemies
7. Approach to the Innermost Cave
8. The Ordeal
9. Reward
10. The Road Back
11. Resurrection
12. Return with the Elixir

In Figure SIII.1 and the table below I relate each of these stages to what I'm calling the Healing Journey, to illustrate the parallels. Without going into each stage of the journey, I wish to point out that one must leave the shoreline of the known or ordinary world and enter a non-ordinary world in which one meets the obstacles and impediments visible here. These obstacles are the deep habit patterns not useful to our growth that block spiritual advancement. Witnessing what is below the surface is an important way to begin to weaken the grip of these deep impressions. But for many, meditation in its formal sense is not accessible or a relatable enough process. By entering the deeper layers and retrieving what is operating beneath our awareness, driving us to act in non-useful ways, ways that could be actually killing us, we can sort out how these deeply rooted patterns work. We can then work with them to untangle the actions they engender from the needs they seek to fill and work to repattern with awareness. In Joseph Campbell's words (Moyers, 1988, dialog#115), "When people find out what it is that's ticking in them, they get straightened out."

In the third and final act of this story arc of the hero's journey, the hero returns to the world renewed and changed. S/he/they now possess knowledge that can be shared with others.

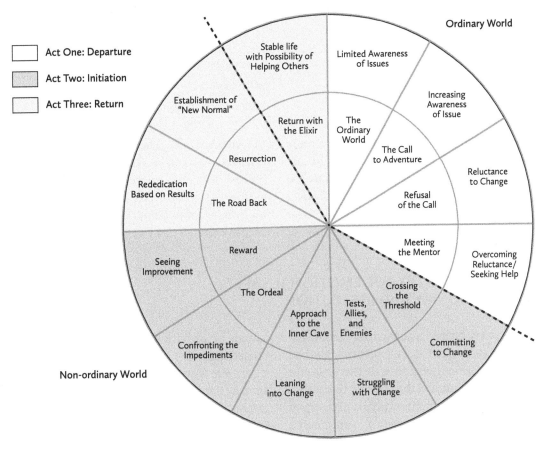

Figure SIII.1 The Hero's Journey of Healing

Hero's Journey and Healing Journey Comparison

The Hero's Journey (Vogler)	The Healing Journey (Schmitt)
Act One: The Ordinary World	
Ordinary World	Limited Awareness of Issue
Call to Adventure	Increased Awareness of Issue
Refusal of the Call	Reluctance to Change
Meeting with the Mentor/Supernatural Aid	Seeking Help
Crossing the First Threshold	Committing to Change
Act Two: The Descent or Initiation	
Tests, Allies, Enemies	Struggling with Change/Road of Trials
Approach to the Inmost Cave	Leaning into Change
The Ordeal	Confronting the Various Impediments
The Apotheosis (The Climax)	
Reward	Seeing Improvement

cont.

The Hero's Journey (Vogler)	The Healing Journey (Schmitt)
Act Three: The Return	
The Road Back	Rededication Based on Results
Resurrection/Master of the Two Worlds	Establishment of "New Normal"
Return with the Elixir/Freedom to Live	Stable Life—Possibility to Help Others

I suppose until yoga therapy becomes a more recognized and established method of healthcare the field will value and promote waking-state scientific evidence to substantiate its efficacy over showcasing personal transformation, which is far less directly measurable but a significant part of the work we offer. The essence of yoga therapy is healing as transformation and this process, as we have seen above, necessitates an experiential journey to states within in which we depart from the waking state (*jagrat*) and travel inward to deeper *koshic* levels of mind and beyond.

CREATING A CONTEXT OF EMOTIONAL SAFETY FOR SELF-INQUIRY AND REFLECTION

Perhaps you've been in a public yoga class, taken a posture as instructed, and surprisingly had a strong emotional response to the pose. Or maybe you've witnessed this happen to another person, seemingly out of nowhere. Often, upon reflection, some life struggle or event can be recalled that has preceded this. Maybe there was some worry or concern that made itself known during class. The body position could have been one of vulnerability like *Matsyasana*, the Fish Pose, or one of fortitude like *Virabhadrasana*, the Warrior Pose. Whatever the case, it appears that the body position demanded the body to move energy in a particular way that brought a torrent of emotion. These feelings may have been held in check while performing the necessary actions of life with little time or space for such processing.

In our work with clients in yoga therapy we may not be able to anticipate every possible response to the work that can potentially arise, but we certainly can work to give options and make the further processing of what comes up as emotionally safe as possible. In doing this we look for the readiness in the person for the work, strive to establish a *sattvic* state within that person, and communicate well and effectively, giving options and supporting autonomy and agency in the individual doing the work. Here are some specifics we can do when working with ourselves and others to create a space for safe introspection to occur.

ESTABLISHING RELATIVE SAFETY IN SUPPORT OF THE INWARD JOURNEY OF TRANSFORMATION

As we provide guidance for our clients to take their own Hero's Journey, we can assure them the path has been tread and is well worth the peril. The journey has been characterized throughout human history as the one taken by each heroic soul in making their way toward meaningfully living their best life. What makes it safe enough to take that first step? How is each person convinced the journey of transformation is worth the effort and discomfort? Is it a greater risk to stay put than to travel?

First and foremost is the readiness of the client. Is the issue ready for attention and is the client ready to change? This naturally involves timing and recognition on the part of the client. When there is readiness, the therapist acts as a facilitator.

As yoga therapists our role can be multifaceted. We can work at all levels and know that work at each one influences all the others. Yet essential to the path of unfolding hidden and overt impediments to becoming more fully who we all truly are is safety during the process of discovery and unfoldment.

This is the safety of trustworthy engagement, of ventral vagal tone, and of being heard and understood. It is the safety of nonjudgmentally holding space for the work to take place, and of the client to have agency in controlling the pace of their own process and being in charge of calling the whole investigation off if they so choose. In keeping with the fact that this is yoga therapy, this safety is founded on the possibility of a higher power positively at work in all our lives.

Supporting and allowing clients to do their own work takes skill and patient practice, but,

in my experience, it yields exceptionally valuable results. It's important to repeat here that self-study is not as fruitful if a *sattvic* state of balanced clarity and discriminative acumen has not yet been established by the client. The foundational practices of yogic breath awareness, balanced *asana* and *vinyasa*, *sattvic* food choices, movement and rest for the client's system, and the steady pervasive expansion of mindfulness in the client's self-reflective capacity are necessary to establish a good enough baseline of clarity and balance within the person seeking the work.

Education may also be needed in terms of how yoga works, its philosophy and psychology, as well as preparation for what to expect when engaging in a natural steady process of self-work. It takes time and patient practice. This may need to be explained, as westerners may be used to more manipulative western interventions that do not engage the patient in the process of self-work and self-discovery.

Below are some safety features for inner work (and really any work) I've found help to create the container for the work so necessary to healing and growth. Please consider having these in place prior to doing the work described in the chapters ahead in this and the following section.

CREATING AN ENVIRONMENT THAT INVITES TRUST AND EASE

It is up to the client to decide whether they feel safe. As yoga therapists, in order to best facilitate and witness their work, we do our level best to create an environment that invites trust. It's up to clients to determine for themselves what that feels and looks like to them. I work to create a safe environment in numerous spoken and unspoken ways. Some arise from my own inner work and development as a seeker on the path. Others are things I do in the space and during our encounter that give the locus of control to my client and meet them as another human

being on the path. I am just the tour guide. It may be that, in some cases, a client will choose to take the practice I outline for them home, set it up in a way that feels safe and doable, and then return to me with a report on whatever they wish to share. In all cases, I'm there for my client in the role of witness-observer and facilitator-guide.

As for my own manner, I hope to show I'm trustworthy by being honestly myself, behaving consistently and reliably with a range of emotional and ethical normalcy. I witness myself and my own responses to the work with discernment, judging when and how I might be useful in its progress. I seek to exhibit good spatial and temporal boundaries and interact in a calm and friendly way. In terms of setting up the environment for deeper work, I do the following:

1. Provide a space that is open and neutral and that has a clear exit.
2. Offer choice to my client so they are clear they are in charge of their own work. They can choose to do or not do, open or not open, change the pace, the direction, or stop at any point. I may also remind them of this as needed as the work progresses.
3. Create a plan for the work with my client so we both know the steps, the timeframe, and what can be anticipated.
4. Have a clear beginning and a clear end to the work, at which point we usually make eye contact and become aware of ourselves in the present moment.
5. Use "I statements" when talking about what I have noticed or observed. This allows the client to be the one who gets to interpret the meaning. I am there with them but am one point of view in the room. I have my background and education to share, but I'm not "God"— although everything is Brahman.
6. After the work has concluded, I offer ways to continue to check in and integrate what they've done into their everyday awareness so it may be usefully applied.
7. Provide any additional educational materials or helpful resources directly related to their work at hand.

CHAPTER 7

Mentally Based Self-Study and the Place of Somatic Inquiry in the Living Tradition of Yoga

My experience of yoga is that it is a practical, systematic discipline, the goal of which is to become aware of my deepest nature. The techniques of yoga, or what I call its vocabulary of practice, are based on the prior experiences of yogis who have achieved this goal. Practicing the techniques is an empirical method of self-study and discovery. At the center of this method is the presumption that a human being has the power to transcend the limiting particulars of personality, personal history, and life events. This transformation occurs in part by finding connection to a powerful source within and allowing it to guide until, at last, realization is complete. The Sanskrit root for yoga (*yuj*), meaning unity or yoke, indicates this purpose.

Not all yoga therapy clients come to us seeking yoga's ultimate goal, nor are all yoga practitioners. Most people come because they want a remedy to some ailment or issue. In yoga therapy practice we mine yoga's richness for applicable elements while honoring its root and ancient goal. For me, yoga philosophy is the framework I hold, and its traditional practices, as I understand them, are its source material. I adapt practices to individual needs accordingly using yoga philosophy, principles, and practices as my source. Sometimes the practice I give is exactly the traditional version. At other times I'll need to modify

it so the person I'm seeking to help can utilize it best for the time being. Their condition will hopefully improve, whereupon they may seek a more ornate or even a more challenging version of the practice going forward.

There are various approaches to yoga, yet a common standard of yoga's main components is represented to a large degree in Patanjali's eight limbs of:

1. *Yama*: codes of self-restraint
2. *Niyama*: self-training observances
3. *Asana*: posture
4. *Pranayama*: expansion of life force through breath
5. *Pratyahara*: withdrawal of the senses
6. *Dharana*: concentration
7. *Dhyana*: meditation
8. *Samadhi*: deep absorption.

The process of yoga practice, whether systematically climbing these limbs or traversing an alternate path, produces in the practitioner increased awareness and discriminative ability. This ability is necessary in discerning what in our lives is beneficial and what is in fact an impediment on our path of awareness and growth. Patanjali's Yoga Sutras discuss impediments as ignorance (Sutras 2.24–25) based in confusion. The path of yoga then provides a remedy, in part through developing the tool of discriminative attention, and in creating conditions for discernment to take place.

ESTABLISHING A STEADY BASE FOR INNER WORK

The Bhagavad Gita (literally "Song of God") is a philosophical poem that, through its story of the battlefield of life, presents a framework for yoga and its goal. Among many other things, it discusses the three *gunas* or qualities of matter, of *tamas*, *rajas*, and *sattva* in relation to what is needed for good discernment. The three *gunas* constitute all of nature, or *prakriti*, in general and the state of the mind in particular. Our thought processes, such as our understanding and judgment, are colored by the qualities of these *gunas*. *Tamas* is characterized by laziness, darkness, dullness; *rajas* by attachment, pain, passion, and restlessness; and *sattva* by clarity, luminosity, and healthy mindedness (*prakasakam anamayam*) (Bhagavad Gita, Verses 14.5–10).

When *sattva* prevails, the mind becomes tranquil. Practices that promote *sattva*, like diaphragmatic breathing, relaxation, meditation, and others that promote ventral vagal tone and autonomic balance, promote this process of distillation in which a person can see clearly. When *sattva* predominates, a person feels mentally expansive and psychologically well despite the ups and downs of life. As the *sattvic* quality increases, the mind gradually becomes skillfully agile and well balanced. The unilluminated, unrefined mind, dominated by *tamas* and *rajas*, however, does not. No amount of talk therapy will have as profound an effect without *sattva* because it provides the somatic basis for clear thinking and discernment.

Here is an example that comes out of the yoga community. In cases of Kundalini activation, arousal or rising, when a *sattvic* state is not attained, the unprepared "gunked-up" body, disorderly energy system, and ungrounded, scattered or dull, confused mind are unable to benefit from this potential state of grace and energy transfiguration. Negative symptoms due to unpreparedness result.

It is through the purification, development, and careful, attentive exercise of the human being's discriminative faculty, or *buddhi*, that self-transformation of any sort moves forward. With a *sattvic* system supporting a well-tuned *buddhi*, the individual is better equipped to sort through the various impressions and experiences that arise on life's transformative journey.

SOMATIC SELF-STUDY AS PART OF A LIVING TRADITION

When I began practicing yoga as a westerner in the United States in the early 1960s I was introduced to a systematic integral approach to yoga in which the outer (*bahir*) practices that address the body and its health served as a preparation and support for its inner (*antar*) practices of mindfulness, self-inquiry, and meditation. Over time, as yoga gained in popularity as a health and fitness modality, I observed a rift between these two aspects, with the inward work being left behind. I'm now beginning to see a return to the integration, with a fresh interest in how these two levels of being—mind and body—psyche and soma—are each experienced within the other.

As yoga is a living tradition, it lives on in me. I honor my teachers and the founders of the lineages with whom I've had the grace and great fortune to study. Some may position yoga as a cultural artifact belonging to a nation. My teachers considered yoga as belonging to humanity. Honoring its roots is to honor a spiritual tradition. Contexting yoga historically one may reference lineages, but these luminary founders and carriers of lineages were more hermits, mendicants, and societal outcasts than governmental dignitaries.

I've spent my life designing ways to stay true to yoga's tenets and purpose while modifying its practices to suit the individual needs of people who seek my help. Over the years I've studied various somatic methods and been exposed to many more. I've found ways to bring the value from these modalities into my practice of yoga. My experience of yoga is that, in its vast inclusiveness, it contains these ways of working within it.

In this section as well you'll see a blend of modern awareness techniques, somatics, and traditional yogic understanding. It's a result of my attempts over the years to meet each person in my practice exactly where they need to be met, and to devise ways in which to work that help them move forward to wholeness. For me, the skill in yoga therapy is in the modification and application of its practices to fit the on-the-spot needs of the individual in an ongoing, developing way. This is not appropriation but evolution. Suiting a practice to an individual for whom a yoga practice would not benefit in its traditional form is not just cutting and pasting yoga into modern life, it's tailoring it with precision, insight, and sincerity, so that it fits and works for someone when off-the-rack would not. Tailoring traditional practice in yoga therapy is an act of compassion not of appropriation.

YOGA'S FRAMEWORK FOR WORKING AT DEEPER LEVELS AND STATES OF BEING

Various models exist within yoga philosophy for understanding the complex nature of human life. In this section on yoga's framework for deeper level work, we'll explore three relevant overlapping concepts: the *koshas*, the states of consciousness, and deeper mental impressions called *samskara* and *vasana*. Two are models of the human experience and the third provides terminology for constellations of feeling, thought, and behavior that this work seeks to explore.

The first such model is the *koshic* model widely used in yoga therapy to distinguish the focus of the therapeutic work. *Kosha*, a Sanskrit word, means covering. In this model, based in Samkhya, the dualistic philosophy that underpins yoga, the human being is considered essentially a spiritual being clothed, you might say, in ever-densifying coverings of matter. The coverings, or *koshas,* are made up of gross to increasingly subtler layers from outside to in. When we refer to inner work, or work at deeper layers, we're referring directly to the interior levels of this model.

THE *KOSHIC* MODEL

Imagine a series of concentric rings like that of a target. The outermost ring represents the most superficial covering or sheath. In this model the outermost ring is the food sheath making up the physical body. Westerners may first be introduced to yoga as a physical wellness practice focused primarily on this level. This outermost sheath is called the *anna maya kosha*, where *anna* literally means food, and *maya* means "is made of." The next level in is the life energy system. The breathing practices, if they are included in a western class, would likely give some exposure to this level. Although breathing is a function of the body, the life force, it is said, rides the breath and can be manipulated directly through breathing practices called *pranayama* (literally "life energy control," or "life energy extension"). In yoga, breathing may also be choreographed to integrate with body position, movement, and even mental activity. Swami Rama has many times said that the breath is the link between the body and the mind, as it is the force that binds the body to the inner layers of being. Experientially, this sheath powers the connection between our outer and inner worlds.

The five *koshas*

1. *Anna maya kosha*—food or physical
2. *Prana maya kosha*—living energy
3. *Mano maya kosha*—sensory-motor mind
4. *Vijnana maya kosha*—discriminative mind
5. *Ananda maya kosha*—blissful or joy-immersed

Traveling inward, the next two layers are distinct aspects of our mental capacity, the *mano maya kosha* and the *vijnana maya kosha*. The more external of these is associated with sensory-motor looping and with the more pedestrian functions of life. *Mano* means mind and refers to the mental screen on which our awareness attends to impressions. Here we interpret and understand sensory input, make mental associations, compare them to memories, plan, and give commands to our body to act. These processes are coordinated here in the mind. I've heard this

layer called the practical mind and the everyday mind. It helps you find your keys.

The next inward level is called the *vijnana maya kosha*, from the Sanskrit root *vi-jna* meaning "to discern, to know rightly, and to understand." This sheath is one of discrimination. It is at this deeper level that we blend the many variables in a decision and at which we may access our intuition and deeper levels of knowing. We may not necessarily call upon this level often throughout our day-to-day life. It is at this deeper level that the development of wisdom, like our capacity to judge what will be beneficial for us, and what will ultimately not serve us in a fruitful way takes place. The term *buddhi*, used earlier, is the power of discrimination in the mind. It is this level at which the *buddhi* exists.

Traveling even further inward there is one more layer described in the Taittiriya Upanishad that may be the most alluring. Called the *ananda maya kosha*, with *ananda* being the Sanskrit word for bliss or joy, it's considered to be the thinnest material layer, and so reflects the light of the luminous eternal self within them all. It may be the level of being described by adepts who find themselves at the doors of transcendence.

Within these five coverings lies the Self or pure consciousness said to be beyond mental conception and thus verbal description. At times this ineffable state is simply referred to as *sat*, *chit*, and *ananda*: *sat* for "existent," *chit* referring to "awareness," and, as we've seen, *ananda* for "bliss." Dwelling in this full awareness (*purna*) while at the same time performing duties in the world through the other *koshas* is yoga's goal.

THE FOUR STATES OF CONSCIOUSNESS

The four states of consciousness are represented by the symbol of Om. This representation is a construct for understanding our experience in terms of a continuum from outward to inward.

It has been related to brain states and states of being moving from alert wakefulness to deep states of absorption.

The Mandukya Upanishad presents the idea

that the primordial sound of Om symbolizes the Self, and that the self exists and is *Brahman* or the universe. It then goes on to discuss the four states of consciousness represented by the expression of Om as A, U, M, and its companionate generative silent state beyond name and form.

The first three states of consciousness in this model are the waking state (*jagrat*), the dreaming state (*svapna*), and the state of deep sleep (*sushupti*).

1. The waking state corresponds to the "A" of AUM and is depicted on the lower curve of the symbol. This state is familiar. We go about our day aware of what we are doing in the world and see this world as real and reliable. Scientific investigation mainly takes place here. This state has to do with outward knowing and the body, so yoga practice that can be proven using the reliable physical data of evidence is accepted.

2. The second state corresponds to the "U" of AUM and is the state of the dreaming mind. It is depicted by the lateral curve on the right side of the Om symbol and is described as inward awareness at the subtle level of being. We have all had dreams and remembered images or feelings from them. Even though dreamed events are not real compared to our waking reality, we may at times find the images or feelings striking and potentially related to some aspects of our waking lives.

3. The third state corresponds to the "M" of AUM and is depicted by the top smaller curve in the symbol. It is the state of deep sleep. In this state the ground of consciousness lies undistracted, yet latent seeds of impressions may still be found here. We do not recall this state while awake, but there may be a sense upon waking that our consciousness has been elsewhere. If we have slept deeply, we may find we've been refreshed in part by our dwelling in this deep sleep state close to the source of our being.

The fourth state is the state of pure consciousness, *turiya* (literally, the fourth). It relates to the *Atman* or Self at the center of the *koshic* rings and serves as the background for all the other states. It is said that a true master has the capacity to dwell in all these states at one time.

HABITS AND PATTERNS (*SAMSKARA* AND *VASANA*)

When we seek to work at deeper layers of being we move into the interior world of mind, which includes patterns of thought, feeling, and subsequent action. In the language of yoga these are sometimes called habit patterns and deep impressions, termed *samskara* and *vasana* respectively. There are many interpretations of these terms. It's beyond the scope of this writing to discuss them at length but I'd like to point to an aspect of habit patterning important to our work. It is the idea of deeply rooted patterns within us. I see the term *samskara* referring more to actions, to habits we enact, and the ruts or groves of actions we do and redo that create a momentum toward continuity. This could be getting up at roughly the same time each day, or having two cups of coffee not one, or going out for a walk at lunch whether you feel like it or not. Some habits are helpful, others not so much. Expectation, creature comfort, and even physiology help us maintain things we repeatedly do.

Still deeper than this, we can become aware of not only the actions we do, but also the constellation of feeling that motivates action. I awaken and feel sluggish and decide I don't like this feeling. The action that may ensue is to have coffee. But prior to the action is noticing how I feel and my judgment or response to what I notice. I may think I have a lot to do today, I've got to get going, and then judge my sluggishness as a negative state, for which coffee is my remedy. If I repeat this process, I may try to avoid all feelings of sluggishness, judging them as bad and a state to get out of as soon as possible. The series of decisions I make to fortify this habit may not even be conscious, or only fleetingly so. It may begin to affect my sleep or ability to calm down and regulate my energy. In this example, I'm talking about an adult. Childhood decisions, made in response to events preverbally, also become part of our patterning, residing way below the surface of awareness. I assign the term *vasana* to these deeper constellations of feelings and responses. They often exist at body level.

MEDITATION AS A BASIS FOR SELF-REFLECTIVE INQUIRY

Formal meditation is a practice that yields a host of skills in the practitioner. Meditation allows us to concentrate in a relaxed way which in turn helps us develop our inner witness-observer, a part of us able to remain relatively objective. As the mind becomes quiet, it's possible to observe its content with increasing clarity. While there are many methods of meditation, the point of the practice is to be able to simply observe the pageant of thoughts without getting caught up in them. The formal practice I teach that is rooted in my tradition involves some preparatory steps that provide a conducive physiological set-up for focusing the mind with minimal distraction. Of course, a clean, well-ventilated, private place that's comfortable enough is optimal as well. The preparatory steps are:

1. physical stillness with the spine vertically aligned
2. relaxation so that each area of the body from head to toe is free of unnecessary activation
3. rhythmic diaphragmatic breathing that allows the breath to be even, smooth, and steady, without pause
4. breath awareness that allows the mind to rest on the steady movement of the breath.

Once these conditions are established, the repetition of a mantra can begin. A mantra is a sound or series of sounds used as the object of focus. A mantra that supports optimal breathing and can be done by everyone is *soham*. The sound "*so*" is recited on inhalation, "*ham*" on exhalation. The sounds are not spoken out loud but repeated mentally. *Soham* mimics, to some degree, the natural sound of breathing, and is translated as "I am That," with "That" being one's Divine nature, or "I am who I am." The practice then continues with gentle effort in keeping the mind focused on repeating the sound. In this practice, over time the sound repetition becomes more automatic and spontaneous.

This practice is the seed of the work ahead. It is the basis of the skill needed in observing what there is in the mind without identifying with it. In self-study or *svadhyaya* we are utilizing the skill that develops, that of being able to step back and look at what our mind is chewing on as a preliminary requirement.

What's next is that we look at the thoughts and impressions. In a more traditional sense, we may focus on discerning whether the thoughts we are noticing are useful or not. This is a direct, cognitive approach of discernment. For instance, I may discover I'm saying repeatedly throughout the day, "Geez oh, you're such a dummy!" whenever I make a mistake, or some result comes from my effort that is unexpected. I may not have ever paid attention to my mental habit of saying this before. But now that I have noticed it I can ask myself if this is something I wish to continue to do.

This is a worthwhile practice with which to engage. We often don't notice thought patterns. And thoughts precede actions. Much can be uncovered in our waking state with this practice. However, some individuals have neither the inclination nor ability to learn a formal meditation practice, let alone stick with it to attain the benefit. For them, the idea of modifying the practice, breaking it into functional pieces that they can employ, is a beneficial way to go. In these cases, practices that bring the client to work with their interior world by turning attention inward but that remain primarily mentally based can be used when resourcing the body more fully and directly is not the right choice for the client at that time.

MENTALLY BASED SVADHYAYA

Introspection, the examination of one's own mental and emotional processes on the part of the client assisted by the yoga therapist, can be a large part of what needs to happen for healing to occur. In facilitating this, we work together to ascertain what habit patterns, behaviors, beliefs, patterns of thinking, and myths to which one subscribes have become impediments to wellness, growth, and attainment of union. There are many ways to introspect and bring what is held within into the clear light (sattva) of reasonable analysis. In the following chapters I will delve more deeply into somatically sourced practices focused on the body. The practices in the rest of this chapter provide an introduction and are a way to develop skill in the process of self-observation. I consider them mentally based as they only draw on the body as one option for where attention may settle. In the somatically sourced practices we'll come to later, awareness is centered in the body throughout the process, with other channels of perception included to embellish the content as it flows into conscious awareness.

CHANNEL AWARENESS

Channel awareness is a practice that arises from meditative and contemplative work, but also references the felt sense of the body. It can help someone recognize that consciousness operates separately from that which it perceives, and that the content of what the mind is focused on is just that—content. It is a practice in paying attention to how information comes into awareness, i.e., through what mode it occurs to us upon the screen of the mind. The body is, of course, the apparatus of our perception, and at times the information we receive is external to us, coming into our awareness through what Samkhya creation theory calls the five entrance senses (jnanendriyas) of seeing, hearing, touching, smelling, and tasting. At other times we sense inside our body (proprioception), noticing what it feels like, feeling how we are moving in space (kinesthesia), or simply how we are feeling generally and overall (interoception). Arnold Mindell has also referred to perception from non-sensory based knowing, calling these modes of awareness the relationship channel and world channel (in Goodbread, 1987, pp. 21–27). I've added an intuitive channel to this mix, for the occasion when something comes like a flash from elsewhere but doesn't seem to arise from one of these known pathways of knowing. I also began noting things that came up as if from a deeper source within me, so I called this channel grace, for lack of a better term. Additionally, I added an interoception channel for when several channels seemed to at once present simultaneously through my body. These developments may not be useful for someone just trying to get the knack of awareness tracking. I use the first ones only when I introduce this work. I eventually made two levels for this. The complex level is often more useful for tracking thematic and behavioral events (see Figure 7.1).

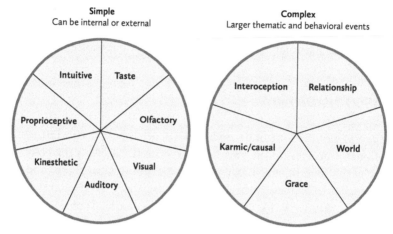

Figure 7.1 Channels of awareness

SOMATIC PRACTICE: Channel tracking

In this practice one becomes aware of the mode in which impressions come into awareness.

1. With these channels in mind, turn inward and become quiet. Allow the mind to focus for a moment on the breath.
2. Then, using a pencil, iPad, or something else on which to write, simply track your attention by marking down on which channel your mind seems to be focused. You can use a simple letter like "V" for visual, "A" for auditory, and the like. There may be inner seeing, like seeing something in your mind's eye, or outer seeing, like seeing the wall before you. Note this distinction if you like.
3. You will not be able to track every quicksilver movement of your mind, but you'll get a rough sketch of its movements.
4. Do this for a set period of time; a few minutes will do at first.
5. Then examine your data. Is there a pattern? Do you cycle through in a similar loop from seeing to feeling to moving and back to seeing? Are there modes of knowing you have, at least in this exercise, avoided? Do you stay in your head and avoid the body entirely? Do you remain inside your body and hesitate to move outward with your sensory perceptions?

Repetitive practice of this exercise can give a person insight into their manner of being without delving into the content of what is on the channel, and so can be a good first step for more internal work. This practice offers a way to observe habitual patterns of perception and attention. It can serve as an opening to deeper exploration as well.

SOMATIC PRACTICE: Stream of consciousness recording

I think of stream of consciousness talking and writing like priming the pump of the mind. It is the opposite of what a traditional meditation teacher wants you to do, which is to return to the mantra and let go of the mental chatter. In this exercise you step back from being attached to the chatter, but allow it to flow. It's a bit like sorting through the trash bin. To do that you have to see what's there so you can see if something may be of value to you. This is similar to Jung's active imagination in which, from a relaxed state, words and images are invited to come into awareness. Recalled dream images can also be used as points of departure for free association. Figures that may occur can be dialogued with, queried, or observed as their action continues—the point being to access the contents of deeper levels of mind as they arise as images, words, feelings, storylines, personifications, or entities. This is not unlike the inner accessing done by artists in their artmaking process. A key to the process is to exert as little influence as possible on the content as it unfolds.

1. Set a time for your exploration. Five minutes is a good starting amount of time.
2. From a relaxed state, bring your attention inward.
3. Notice the first thing that comes to mind and then follow that. It may be that you see or speak to yourself or hear an external sound like the tick of a clock. Record your experience either by saying what it is or writing it down. You may also notice bodily sensations or have the urge to move.
4. Continue to follow the flow of your experience, capturing what you can and writing it down or saying it.
5. When the time is up, bring your awareness to the external space around you. Make eye contact with anyone else working with you. Pause.
6. Now have a look at what was captured. See what catches your interest. Is there anything new? Does anything strike you as significant? Notice what you notice.

SPATIAL TABLEAU WORK

Another activity for bringing into the light of awareness what may be at first hidden from view is the act of setting a stage or making a tableau. This relies on our sense of space, a topic covered earlier. That space is expressive is an important feature, and that space is the place in which we live our lives means we embody it as well. Creating a picture in space, either on paper or by setting a stage with objects or figures, like a freeze frame of a scene from a play, will give information about interactional relationships based on spatial relationships in that field. Once the tableau or stage is set, the person who made it can then reflect on the felt meaning the set-up engenders. We respond somatically to spatial features like proximity, size, and volume. Our impression may symbolize something to us, and at the same time we can have a visceral, precognitive reaction to how the space is being used and inhabited. Observing the use of space can give information about deeper aspects of what it is we are perceiving within and around us.

MAKING A TABLEAU OR DIAGRAM

You can certainly start off by making a simple diagram or image of a setting in which you function and then reflect upon it. A client once brought up that she felt anxious at her job as a nurse in a doctor's office. She felt constantly on edge and this was negatively affecting her blood pressure. At my request, she began to describe her day, which involved moving from the reception area to the many offices and exam rooms. I had a sense that her use of space was in some way important to her dilemma, so I asked her to make a quick sketch of the office layout (see Figure 7.2). Since we were in my office, I opened my cabinet of small figures and gestured to her that if she wished she could use them.

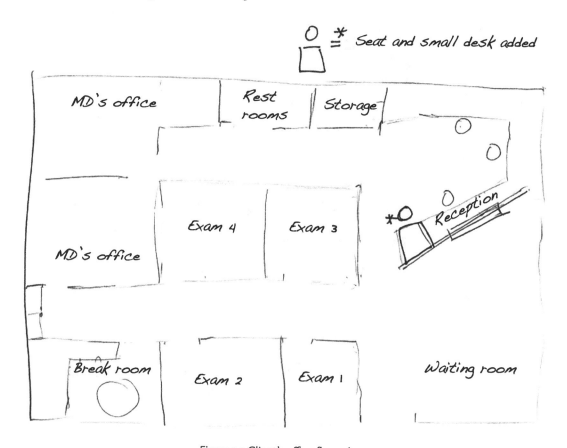

Figure 7.2 Client's office floor plan

She created a diagram of the office space in which the receptionist and each practitioner had their own cubicle or office with at minimum a desk and chair. She then placed a figure representing each co-worker in their spot. I asked her where she was in the space. She held a small stone figure of a sea turtle and said, "Nowhere. I'm always on the move. There is no one place for me. The only place I stop moving is when I have lunch in the break room, which is a common space shared by everyone." We began to work toward a practical solution that involved assigning her an office chair and a small but sufficient portion of the reception desk for her to call her own. What ensued were more assertions of her right to be and be comfortable in her work and life.

SOMATIC PRACTICE: Making a tableau or diagram

You can work with a real setting as in the example above or see how you would create a spatial image of some problem you are addressing, a family dynamic, or any other sort of depiction. The main idea is to get what is in your mind out into space so you can see it, respond, and learn more about yourself.

1. Choose a topic. Identify the parts in it. You may add more parts later but choose a few for starters.
2. Outline the space you will use. An open, uncluttered studio is great for this, but a blank piece of printer paper will suffice. If you need to, section off an area of the space you'll use with nothing in it so it can become a blank canvas for what you'll make. (You can make an outline of the space with resistance bands or whatever you have.)
3. If you're in the scene, decide if you will place yourself first or last. Then begin to place the elements of the scene in the space you've made. Try not to think too much, just allow your body to move based on your experience of the topic and its parts.
4. If you've chosen to place yourself last, do so.
5. Now step back and observe your reaction as you look at the scene. You may find you need to adjust a thing or two, but after that, leave it alone and simply observe it and your responses.
6. If you like, jot them down, record them verbally on your iPhone, or, if someone is with you, share your impressions verbally with them. If you would like, feel your body and allow it to move freely in any way that occurs in response to the tableau you've made.

ROLE PLAY

At times what may emerge from tableau work are two sides of an issue. It could be a decision to make: whether or not to purchase a big-ticket item, whether or not to have knee surgery, whether or not to host Thanksgiving Dinner this year, or to forgive a significant other. In creating a special diagram of how you feel about your relatives after your dad's death, you may discover hard feelings for someone you didn't realize you were harboring because of the placement on the page. Wherever the schism lies, setting up two or more positions in space, either evolving from the tableau or by simply using two chairs, you can take on one role and then the other to flesh out the dialogue between the parts. You might even record what you say, or have someone there with you to do just that.

This can remain a deeply embodied experience of trying on the body language posture and subsequent feeling state of one position and then the other, or it may simply be sourced from the words and images residing in your mind. Two hands, two pens, one held in each hand, or simply turning in opposite directions when you embody and speak each point of view can serve as spatial orientation for this work.

As above, the point here is to flesh out what is revealed by the tableau and allow each part to share its perspective. We will return to this more fully in the upcoming somatic *svadhyaya* section in Chapter 9.

CHAPTER 8

Framework for Somatic Practices for Self-Inquiry and Reflection

INNER WORK STRUCTURE

As we turn toward the practices that begin to explore deeper levels and states of being, I'd like to set out a structure for understanding how the pieces fit together, as I am drawing from the yoga tradition and beyond it. This is not only to justify the somatic work ahead, but also to help you navigate the way I'm presenting it. The structure relies on some variation of these four parts: the container, the witness-observer, the mode of perception, and the flow of content.

CREATING THE CONTAINER

The first necessary area for consideration is what I'll call the safe container. It usually consists of these elements:

1. Enough space in which to do the practice (whatever form it takes) free from distractions.
2. A "judgment-free zone," usually enacted by the presence of a witness-observer who tries their level best to be non-judgmental while observing the person whose work is happening, as well as their own response to it. At times one may work alone, in which case one's own internal witness-observer role is called upon. This can be developed through consistent practice and makes a good basis for further, more interactive, therapeutic interactions.
3. A timeframe in which the work takes place, with a clear beginning and ending.
4. A plan for the work taking place so that all participants are clear and can engage within their sense of comfort and autonomous control.
5. An agreement to follow the set-up and plan for the work. This may include making eye contact when coming out of the work, abiding by the timeframe, owning one's own experience, and commenting accordingly, if that is part of the plan.

THE WITNESS-OBSERVER STANCE

If you practice meditation in the yoga tradition, you are likely familiar with the witness-observer stance. To take this stance you simply attempt to observe the flow of the movement of thoughts in your mind without being disturbed or attached to any of them. There are more elaborate instructions, but this is the essence. The practice itself is known to weaken one's attachment to the content of the thoughts, giving greater ability to step back, pause, and consider before acting. Being able to separate conscious awareness from what is appearing on the screen of the mind gives us more control. With practice we begin to understand that who we are is different from the thought occurring at any moment. The quiet focus of witnessing also helps create the container mentioned above. The person doing the work may gain a sense of being held and seen by a nonjudgmental presence. This often allows for greater depth of work to arise, with the witness providing a sense of security and benevolence associated with the self in its most gracious form.

THE MODE OF PERCEPTION

The mode of perception is the vehicle of that which we are paying attention to. Arnold Mindell, the creator of Processwork, calls these modes channels of experience (Mindell, 2011). They include our five senses and awareness of our movement. Some inner work techniques may work with only one channel, like seeing on the visual channel. They may keep the focus on the auditory channel, as in mantra repetition, so that something appearing on a different channel, say an ache in the back, is identifiable as a distraction. Hearing something other than the mantra, such as a dog barking or child crying, is also a disturbance to the practice being attempted. The mode, then, is *how* what we perceive is coming in.

THE FLOW OF CONTENT

In various translations of the Yoga Sutras *chitta* is defined as the "mind-stuff" or storehouse of impressions. In yoga philosophy the *chitta* is considered one of four aspects of the mind called the *antah karana* (literally the inside (thing) that functions). In some interpretations the *chitta* is considered synonymous with western psychology's unconscious, of which there is an individual and a collective. So, certainly, the flow of the mind's content overall will contain some of what has been stored as well as more superficial sense impressions in the moment. Right now, the sun is shining in my eyes. I perceive this on the screen of my mind and remember when I was on vacation lying on the beach with the sun in my eyes, a memory sourced from my *chitta*, or storehouse of impressions. So the flow of content is that which appears to my conscious awareness.

When learning to meditate, the content of the mind is not the focus, rather the focus is learning the skill of stepping back and not jumping on the train of thoughts. Sometimes when meditation is taught it has seemed to me as if thoughts are considered trash to be thrown in the garbage pail. I believe the point of this disregard was to practice letting them go. Still, we can sort through "the rubbish" of our thoughts. As we do, we can sort out what may be useful from what is not. There may be inconsequential superficial impressions mixed in with deeper, older ones. We can learn about ourselves through this kind of introspective process, with witnessing as an underlying skill.

ENTERING THE DEEP

At times it may be useful to invite the client to investigate information held at deeper levels of being. I find this particularly necessary when someone is stuck in a detrimental behavior they can't seem to change. Lifestyle, thought, breathing, and emotional habits are often deep patterns interwoven into our concept of identity. They serve a purpose, although they may have outworn their usefulness long ago. Replacing these patterns can be a straightforward path, but most often when a client is stuck or struggling these patterns are the opposite of straightforward and easy to change. This for me is a main area in which I believe yoga therapy can help a person change. Because these levels are not a normal part of waking state and day-to-day reality it can be helpful to find ways to support and facilitate the client in opening into deeper realms. This must be done, of course, with the utmost safety in place and with readiness and willingness on the part of the client.

Rudolph Ballentine, in the introduction to *Radical Healing* (Ballentine, 1999), asserts that healing is transformation that relies on awareness and our connection to a larger whole. When we are faced with a health challenge, we have the opportunity to enter a process of enlargement of identity. We may be forced to leave behind the patterns and ways of being that got us to this moment. In doing so we face the unknown. This is a universal situation for growth. We depart what is and what is known for the open seas of adventure. Meeting our health challenges with awareness and curiosity allows us to face them as an archetypal mythic journey. As we let go of what was and enter the unknown, we embark on a Hero's Journey, clinging only to our own initiative and developing inner wisdom.

A HISTORICAL PERSPECTIVE: THE ASCLEPION HEALING SANCTUARIES

The value of looking below the surface and working to understand the deeper themes of someone's life is an important feature in healing. We have the work of Freud and Jung and many others in western psychology to thank for the analyst's couch. Prior to Hippocrates, the father of contemporary western medicine, we have the Asclepions, who relied on departure into the dream state as the nexus of cure.

The roots of healing and medicine in ancient Greece lie in religion and spirituality. Asclepius, the Divine Physician, was worshiped as a god, and supplications were made to him for healing. Healing sanctuaries called Asclepions were established throughout Greece, usually in settings of awe-inspiring natural beauty.

There, physician-priests practiced a kind of spiritual healing centered around dream therapy on patient-pilgrims. The preliminary treatment was Katharsis, or purification consisting of cleansing baths and purgations, accompanied by a cleansing diet, lasting several days. Then offerings and rites were performed. From there the patient entered the *Abaton*, or dream incubation chamber, for one or more nights, to receive a healing dream. If the patient-pilgrim was lucky, he would be healed directly in the dream state, otherwise he was told what to do to cure the illness or affliction. The physician-priests at the Asclepions were master dream interpreters who would divine the treatment to be followed from the patient's account.

From the ancient Greek Asclepions comes the concept of the healing sanctuary, the descendants of which are the health spas popular throughout Europe. It's difficult to imagine that Freud and Jung had no knowledge of these practices as they developed their modern psychological theories.

Hippocrates' establishment of medicine as a rational science freed it from magic, religion, and the supernatural. Perhaps this was because it was thought that Hippocrates' father was a physician-priest in the Asclepion at Kos, where young Hippocrates got his first practical experience and training in the art of healing.

HOW SOMATIC PRACTICE FITS INTO YOGA'S INNER WORK OF SELF-STUDY (*SVADHYAYA*)

At times the solution to a complaint is simple. A postural habit is remedied with strengthening, stretching, and movement repatterning. At other times there is more to the story. Areas of the body that appear to be "offline," or are presenting symptoms, have reason for doing so. Presenting issues may reveal ingrained strategies for living and ways of feeling so deeply hidden in family of origin and cultural myths that they're invisible—at first. Yoga includes the whole person: body, energy, emotion, mind, and spirit. When working with one level of being, other levels of being may be involved.

A portion of my approach to yoga therapy is a section I call Spanda® Self-Reflective Inquiry™ or Spanda® SRI™. It includes a variety of ways to work with the inner *koshic* layers beyond the physical and energetic. Some of these ways stay more in the mental realm in that they're not sourced directly from the body and its many signals as impetus for the work. Other avenues we'll explore are directly sourced there. I call this somatically based self-study (*svadhyaya*), or simply somatic *svadhyaya*.

Svadhyaya is an aspect of *niyama*, one of Patanjali's eight limbs of yoga. A compound Sanskrit word, it combines *sva* and *adhyaya*. *Sva* means "one's own" and *adhyaya* translates as "a lesson, lecture, chapter, or reading." Therefore, *svadhyaya* literally means "one's own reading." *Svadhyaya* is also a compound word that combines *sva* with *dhyaya*, which means "meditating on." *Svadhyaya*, then, also refers to contemplation, meditation, self-reflection, to make inquiry into the nature of one's own self.

In traditional circles *svadhyaya* is interpreted as study of scriptures combined with practice in applying the principles taught in them to life. This is similar to the practice of *Lectio Divina* in the Christian tradition. In this practice scripture is read and reflected on, with time for prayer and deep guidance.

If we consider the body as a sort of gospel or source of direct teaching, then the reading of the living body and its supportive energy grid can be considered a form of *svadhyaya*. This would be the body as text, you might say. How is the body like a text? It can be read and interpreted. We look for meaningful information all the time when it comes to the body—signs and symptoms tell us what is going on, how we are challenged in some way, what illness, injury, or chronic imbalance is limiting us. We blush when embarrassed, our pupils dilate when we're afraid. These responses are automatic, and no amount of wishing is going to stop them from revealing our inner state.

Because of this, somatic *svadhyaya* can give us information about our deeper patterning that is often not apparent, precisely because it is hidden from view.

Western medicine will give a heart attack survivor a series of preventative medications going forward from that point. However, the detrimental lifestyle habits like poor diet, smoking, and lack of exercise, along with the stressful emotional patterning of that person—unless addressed—will remain intact. The underlying and often unexamined beliefs and ways of moving through life held by that individual keeps these lifestyle choices and patterns in place.

Lifestyle advice abounds in practically every medium in the modern world. TV shows, social media ads, and healthcare newsletters will give ten things to do for practically any condition. If information is so plentiful and readily available, why then are people so unhealthy? Is changing a lifestyle habit or foundational aspect of one's operating system more than a straightforward path?

Once an undesirable pattern of behavior or impediment is discovered and identified, the various approaches to addressing change can be sorted into two main groups. One is to focus on the goal and find ways to reach it. This approach assumes that there are no icebergs of difficulty lying hidden at deeper layers. If this straightforward approach is not effective, then focusing on the impediment to change may unfold the information and understanding that can then lead to the desired change—or even to something entirely unexpected (see Figure 8.1).

Two Approaches to Change for the Better	
Focus on the Goal	Focus on the Impediment to the Goal
Move Toward What is Wanted	Remove or Dismantle and Reintegrate the Impediment
What you seek is seeking you—Rumi	*What is in your way is your way*—Anonymous

Figure 8.1 Two approaches to change for the better

Working with impediments will most often involve the deeper *koshic* layers, because the impediments are often lodged in the deep impressions, feeling states, patterns of perception, and interpretation of meaning rooted and operational in the causal and subtle bodies.

This content or material is organized symbolically. This is why working with storytelling, artmaking, self-inquiry, and myth are such valuable means for uncovering what is operating in someone at deeper levels.

In many cases, however, this way is not fully informed until the body has its say. This is because our bodies store information at a non-verbal level. There is a somatic narrative that needs to be revealed and received by conscious awareness. Our experiences are lived somatically through our sensory and interoceptive systems, i.e., awareness of internal states of comfort and discomfort. We can mine the body for its held impressions. This involves careful attentive work and the development of the client's *buddhi* in a stable, *sattvic* environment with the caring presence of a well-trained witness-guide.

CHAPTER 9

Somatic *Svadhyaya* Practice: Self-Inquiry with the Body as Source

In the yoga tradition from which this work evolved there is a saying: all the body is in the mind but not all the mind is in the body. To me this means that the mind can attend to the body —we're capable of feeling into the body deeply with awareness, and attend outside of it, paying attention to our environment. We can also imagine things that aren't really there, remember things, and think abstractly.

In what I call the mentally based or mentally sourced *svadhyaya* in Chapter 7, we're working with the mind. In those cases information from the body is merely one of many options from which the mind can draw impressions. Here, with what I'm terming somatic *svadhyaya*, the mind remains focused on the body's signals as the wellspring of information to be developed, filled in, and worked with.

MINING THE BODY FOR MEANING

We can explore the body's nonverbal signals for potential hidden meaning. If we consider the body's positions, movements, and what we feel in our body to be avenues of communication from levels of self not ordinarily available to our waking state, they may be considered signals. Some of these signals may carry valuable information into consciousness. This process is like mining the earth to discover treasures of great value held within it. Symptoms, pain, and persistent annoyances may be explored and unfolded through a guided process that has the potential to reveal important information specific to our unique strategies for living.

If we're interested in learning more about things within us that, despite our best efforts, impede us, we can look at the information appearing in our channels of perception. As we've seen in the previous chapter, we could explore information occurring through inward or outward seeing, inward or outward hearing, through taste and smell, and through our intuition. We might even consider uncanny synchronistic events as information coming to awareness on a cosmic channel. On the body level, information may appear as body sensations, emotions, pain, unintentional movements like twitches, and physical effects like sweating, feeling hot or cold, blushing, and other types of things we don't necessarily control. If we construe the information gleaned from these signals as messages from a larger framework of self, we can listen to it and consider the meaning it may have for us. This can become part of the expansion of consciousness described by yogis over the millennia.

Through this work we literally can expand our definition of self by accepting things that our ego-identity initially finds unacceptable. When we include what, from a narrower perspective, we may at first consider un-includable, we open to a larger framework than our personality construct. By doing so, we participate in the interconnected field of being that is us and that also surrounds us. Expanding our ego-identity from its narrow self-view to include aspects heretofore excluded can be freeing, healing, empowering, and transformative.

This process of transformation is deeply Tantric. Tantric teacher Rudolph Ballentine describes the buildup of energy through *tapas* or containment. The strategy involves letting a natural or habitual urge (*spanda shakti*) build energy by denying its outlet (*tapas*) while remaining present and identified in one's witness consciousness of what is experienced. He describes the transformation that can happen if the energy collecting is not automatically expended (Ballentine, 1999, pp. 447–453). He discusses this phenomenon at the energetic level (*prana maya kosha*). In our work, we'll consider it at the levels of the food sheath (*anna maya kosha*) and the mental sheaths (*mano maya kosha* and *vijnana maya kosha*) as well. Doing this adds a dimension of working with signals, figures, and personal and cultural myths found individually and universally in our psyche, dreamlife, and creative imaginings.

SOMATICALLY BASED *SVADHYAYA*

If we consider the body to be a nonverbal medium through which deeper levels of self—holding deep impressions and patterning—can communicate to our waking conscious state, we can explore the body's signs, signals, movements, and sensations for potential meaning.

If we consider the body's positions, movements, and other observables to be avenues of communication from levels of self not ordinarily available to our waking state awareness, they become signals. Some of these can be observable by others, such as body position and tone of voice. Other signals are observable only to that person, as in interoceptive body sensing. These signals carry valuable information into consciousness. Symptoms, pain, persistent annoyances can be unfolded through a guided therapeutic process to reveal information that may be below consciousness yet operating within us in hidden ways.

We'll explore interrelated methods of somatic *svadhyaya* through the body. The first presents a continuum that provides an accessible way to enter this work from the practice of *asana*, a yoga practice familiar to most people. The next three forms mine the body more directly for information not forthcoming by non-somatic means. They are called Dreaming in Movement, Myofascial Activation™, and Somatic Access Tracking™.

THE FORM-TO-FORMLESS CONTINUUM OF PRACTICE IN THREE STAGES

This practice is a good introduction to paying attention to what the body is saying and easing into allowing that content to come forward. The amount of leeway taken to explore the felt sense of one's body's inner impulses and responses to a yoga *asana* is the theme of the continuum described below.

A continuum is a spectrum of variations that blend from one extreme to the other. On one end of this continuum are positions we put the body into to the best of our ability. The forms or the yoga poses are learned and then performed with attention to getting them right by attending to their formal spatial features. We try to do the yoga practice as exactly as possible, like a gymnast who attempts to execute a move for a perfect score. This is the goal-oriented side of the continuum, and it gives a particular experience to the practitioner. On the opposite end, the formal features of the practice are absent, and the practice becomes attending solely to the body's sensations and the movements they elicit. In some circles this is called the impulse to move. What you do physically on this far end of the continuum is not planned. The practice is centered on observing the impulses that emerge and allowing them to express through the body in each moment. You simply allow an impulse to play out its *spanda* by following its energy as it emerges into physical movement.

SOMATIC PRACTICE: Stage 1: Insight from embodying the form

This is the typical approach to the practice of yoga postures you might find in a yoga class today—but with the added intent of learning more about myself through my body. I'm interested not only in doing the pose correctly to gain its benefits, but also in what ways I may not be able to do the pose correctly.

To do this practice, pay attention to body sensations as a way to gauge how fully your body in this particular moment is able to embody the form of the pose, while remaining aware of your capacity. Merge as fully as your capacity allows into the form of the posture. From this you'll accrue the benefits of the pose in terms of energy flow, stretching and/or strengthening, pattern of breathing, and other perks specific to the pose you've chosen. In addition, once in the pose, notice anything about your practice of the pose that does not seem to be fully doing the pose. Simply make a note of it. You can do any pose you like. As an example, I've chosen one of my favorites, Triangle Pose or *Trikonasana*. Please modify the pose in any way to suit your needs.

1. Begin by standing sideways on your mat with feet hip-distance apart. Pay attention to your breath and relax any extraneous tension. Tune into your body.
2. Step your feet wide apart with heels aligned to each other.
3. Turn your right leg out from your hip to the side to around 90 degrees so the toes are pointing to the top of your mat.

Check that the center of your right knee is aligned with the center of your right ankle.
4. Pivot your left leg inward slightly from your hip, to about a 45-degree angle.
5. Raise your arms to your sides at shoulder height, so they're parallel to the floor, palms down.
6. On an exhalation, reach through your right hand in the same direction as your right foot is pointed and fold at your right hip to bend to that side. Keep your right ear, shoulder, and knee on the same plane, not allowing your torso to drop forward. Turn your left palm forward as you reach that arm upward.
7. Rest your right hand on your right shin, or if you like your ankle. You can also place this hand on a block or a chair seat.
8. Look upward, forward, or downward depending on your balance needs and neck comfort.
9. Activate to maintain the pose by pressing down through the outer edge of the left foot. Expand equally through both sides of the torso while you reach the tailbone toward your left heel. Widen through the arms.
10. Hold for a few breaths or to your comfortable capacity.
11. Before you come up, make a note of anything not fully participating in the pose. Is your hamstring tight and preventing your deepness? Is the arm drifting forward

instead of up? Notice what, if anything, is not fully allowing you to get into or maintain the pose comfortably. This is the content making itself known to you. It is literally what is in the way, that is the way.

12. To come out, inhale and push through the right heel as you bring your torso upright, lowering your arms. Turn the feet forward and step together to notice the effect of the practice before beginning the opposite side.

Now make note of what, if anything, may have prevented you from fully embodying the form of the pose you chose to do. This is where the information lies. At this stage we simply note that there is information available. Because at this stage, we're just bringing into view the fact that there may be content in the body worth further investigation, it's a good point of entry for somatic *svadhyaya* work.

SOMATIC PRACTICE: Stage 2: Dialoguing with the form

This stage moves away from attempting to fit into the form of the pose and moves us toward being comfortable with the content that arises when doing so. I like using the seated head-to-knee pose, *Janu Shirshasana*, for this exercise, but please feel free to use any pose you like.

With this blend of outer direction and inner allowance, we begin to follow the body's signals as we perform a pose. Here we no longer simply acknowledge that there is information in our body, we begin to allow it to come forward.

1. Let's begin by sitting with your left thigh rotated laterally with that knee bent and foot against the opposite inner leg wherever you are most comfortable. The right leg extends forward along the floor.
2. Sitting tall, inhale the arms overhead, and with a long spine tilt from the hips, if possible, forward over the extended leg.
3. When you are comfortably tilting forward, feeling a stretch along the back of the right leg, allow the arms to come down on either side of the leg.
4. Notice what parts of your body you must

actively exert to maintain this pose. For instance, notice that you must exert some action in the inner thigh to medially rotate the right leg into this position. Allow it to relax and roll outward. Then bring it back.

5. See what other aspects of the pose you can allow to release or move while still basically doing the pose.
6. Allow yourself to play with moving out of your version of the full pose and back into it with different body parts such as the spinal reach and head position, the arms, the bent leg, etc. You might even create a *vinyasa* (posture-based movement sequence) from your exploration, by starting in the pose and then moving with one part or another away from the pose and then back to it!
7. When you are no longer interested in what you are doing, come out of the pose. Lie in *Shavasana* and notice what you notice. What did you learn? How do you feel? What is new about your experience of this posture?

SOMATIC PRACTICE: Stage 3: Departure into movement

In this stage you use the yoga pose as a point of departure into movement that may or may not return to the starting point. The focus here now shifts toward following *spanda*, the inner drive to move. This is like free association in movement, beginning from some place you know. You can set a time for the exploration; from a minute to five minutes is a good start.

1. Begin in a pose you choose or start in a standing side bend (*Ardha Chandrasana*). Hold the pose as long as you like, and when you come out pay attention to what the body wishes to do. You may find yourself coming upright, or instead rolling forward into a forward bend, dropping to hands and knees, or something else. From there just continue to notice what it is the body feels like it would like to do. If you are an experienced practitioner of yoga, this may be one of the ways you practice, by simply following your body's impulses for a time.

2. If you've set a time, come to a point of closure when the time is up. If not, allow your body to move freely according to its need and inner impulse until there is a moment of pause that feels for the time being, complete. Then come out of the practice.

3. Stand, sit, or lie down for a few moments to notice the effect of practicing this way. What did you do that was new? What did you discover? How do you feel? For whom might this be of use?

DREAMING IN MOVEMENT

Certainly, everyone who practices yoga on a regular basis has from time to time let go of the form of a posture and moved in response to body sensation. This could be to adjust the pose to greater or lesser intensity. It could be moving a body part or area in response to sensation brought to awareness by the body's position in a pose, or by any number of things.

In typical practice sessions, information that arises in response to the practice—whether on the body sensation level, an exclamation of "ouch," or a quicksilver visual image—is not attended to or followed. Usually, our conscious intention is to remain steady and comfortable (*sthira sukham asanam*) in the pose.

However, for the sake of self-study, what if, instead of staying put in the practice, we allowed our body to depart from the practice and follow the impulse, image, or sensation to learn more? What if we went into instead of away from what has come up for us?

In traditional yoga, allowing movement to happen from a spontaneous impulse is sometimes called a *kriya*. The term *kriya* has other meanings as well. In western circles of movement inquiry allowing for spontaneous movement has been called automatic movement, to parallel the trance-like state of automatic writing. Dreaming in Movement is allowing the body to move freely and spontaneously with relaxed awareness. The purpose is to allow what is within into the conscious stream of awareness. Dream-like imagery, feelings and feeling states, figures, and other information from beyond the conscious waking state are then witnessed.

The information that arises can then be

journaled, drawn, analyzed, used in artmaking, or simply allowed to serve as catharsis. What comes up may hold the key to thought or

behavioral difficulties, the causes of which lie hidden with the deep and latent impressions of the body-mind.

HOW TO DO DREAMING IN MOVEMENT

This practice, and the ones that follow, come from experimentation with self, students, and clients over the past 30 or so years. I've been exposed to several somatic, dance, and healing arts forms, and you may see elements of them I've adapted to this work. For instance, a practice from the realm of the contemplative arts and dance therapy called Authentic Movement uses extemporaneous movement and witnessing, in dyads primarily and in group forms. This practice is adapted from it but is not a replica in that we are specifically working to elicit information from deeper levels of being within this therapeutic context as a form of self-inquiry. In Authentic Movement one is freely open to what might arise. Also, movement improvisation can be a rich and enjoyable form of performance. However, the intention of it is performance. In this work we're referencing the body so that we can learn from the mind that is in the body—from the consciousness that embodies our living tissues.

Movement is often a channel of awareness underutilized in modern culture. We sit and

type and read and watch on screens and, when we do move, it is usually structured. We follow the directions of a yoga teacher in class, execute a *kata* (choreographed form) in a martial art so the movements become automatic, or move with intention to score a goal on the field of play. Yet rarely do we simply allow our body to move freely from an inner impulse.

In Dreaming in Movement the practitioner waits for an impulse to move that arises from sensation or impulse in the body. The impetus could be pain, or emotion, or response to the comfort or discomfort of the starting position. From this start, the practitioner pays attention to the body's feelings and signals and continues to move according to what presents itself. The impulse to move is generative but, after that, other channels of perception come into view and a scene or memory comes into play. The practitioner stays internally focused and allows for movement to continue in response to what is occurring, keeping the felt sense in the body as impetus.

SOMATIC PRACTICE: Dreaming in Movement

This practice can be done alone if one has experience with witnessing. If not, it can be done with another person who shares the role of witness-observer. Both must agree to witness with dispassion. If practicing alone, be sure to establish an internal witness-observer within yourself. One way to get a sense of this is to place some object in the space such as a candle, flower, sacred image, or the like as a reminder.

1. Set a time for the practice; five to ten minutes is good for a first time. Agree to come out and become aware of the here and now when the time is up.
2. Make a safe space by roping off an area or using only the space on a carpet or in some other way designating a clear and empty space for your use.
3. Close your eyes or keep an internal focus. If you make large, fast movements, open

your eyes to make sure you don't hit any objects nearby.

4. Begin in a position that invites movement, rather than something that makes it harder to start moving. For instance, stand or walk to begin rather than lying in *Shavasana*.

5. Wait for an impulse to move or move in a different way, and then allow your body to go with that. Continue to allow your experience to unfold, exerting as little control over what you do as possible.

6. Remain internally focused, following the impulses as they arise for the entire time set. There may be periods of movement and of stillness.

7. When time is up, bring your awareness to the present moment and notice the space around you. Come out of the dream. If working with another person, make eye contact.

8. If you like, take a moment to share any of your impressions, the storyline, or discoveries by writing them down, drawing, or talking with your witness-observer. Over time you'll collect a number of impressions that may add up to something meaningful that you have been curious about.

SPANDA® MYOFASCIAL ACTIVATION™ (SPANDA® MA™)

Spanda® Myofascial Activation™ is a technique to specifically address myofascial trouble spots or trigger points. Trigger points are hyperirritable nodules in skeletal fascia that are tender and that when compressed may produce referred pain. This practice is specifically designed for places in the body not easily remedied by stretching, massage, or a few minutes of foam rolling. Rather it is for areas of persistent discomfort and tightness that haven't been caused by specific injury, especially if an emotional component is suspected. These types of tender spots are good candidates for this work. This technique can be done without an enduring trigger point as the focus. The way to do that will also be discussed below.

SOMATIC PRACTICE: Spanda® Myofascial Activation™

You will need to find a prop or several items that will give you the starting position of elevating the body area chosen for the work, in which the trigger point can be isolated as the high point of the body with the rest of the body draping from it in a relaxed manner. Rolled yoga blankets, small rollers, Gertie or other soft inflatable mini exercise balls, or bolsters can be used. Feel free to be creative in what you find to create the effect of the trigger point being a high point. I have used packing tape to tape beach toweling into the "right" shape for this. Bheka makes a teardrop-shaped small support that is inflatable and so it can serve this purpose for several body areas.

1. Set a time limit for the practice. Ten minutes is a good starting amount of time. If you like, you can have someone with you to again act as an external witness-observer.

2. Choose the spot you wish to investigate and then do some relaxation to reduce the overall tone of the body so the focal nodule can be more clearly felt.

3. Determine how you will place the body area in which the nodule is located facing

upward toward the ceiling. The rest of the body needs to drape comfortably from this high point. You need to be comfortable enough for this work and the focus to be on the nodule. So play around with the right position for you. For instance, when I work with a spot on the outside of my hip, I place the side of my pelvis onto a bolster and let the rest of my body drape to the floor. To isolate the spot even more, I'll place the Bheka prop only one-third inflated on top of the bolster and rest on the side of my pelvis with the nodule facing up.

4. So as not to create too much of a signal of pain, allow the body's weight to fall so the fullest stretch on the nodule is slightly *tangential*. If the center of the nodule or area of pain is the bull's eye of a target, center the nodule onto one of the outer rings of the bull's eye. This will bring up the somatic signal from the nodule without taking you into a higher than useful pain level. You want to have some sensation you can work with, without eliciting a level of pain that you want to get away from. If you are already at an acute level without even positioning the nodule, please wait until your pain has subsided to do this technique. If you're not working with an enduring trigger point, locate an area of high tension or nagging stiffness and create a position of the body to stretch that area, but not to its fullest. If a full stretch is an eight of a scale of ten, stretch the area to a sensation of five or six.

5. Focus inward. Relax as much as possible and wait for signals to appear on the mind-screen in the various channels of awareness. If you are comfortable enough to close your eyes, do so. You may see an image, hear a sound, feel more, or begin to move. Just keep allowing whatever arises to come into your field of consciousness.

6. Use tangential stimulation. If there is not much information readily available, begin to move in such a way that the path of weight bearing crosses the nodule on a tangential path. You want to feel the nodule activate with feedback, but not max out on the pain. This is so you can "mine the body area" for information through the awareness channels. Move in such a way as to feel sensation on a tangent nearby but not crossing the nodule.

7. Capture what comes up. If you are doing this alone, have a notebook, recorder, or something to capture the fleeting subtle images, sounds, feeling tones, and insights that come as you move. A fuller recollection or gestalt may arise. If someone is with you, you can speak these impressions to them while they note them down for you.

8. Stop, pause, or rest at any point in the process.

9. To transition out of the practice, slowly come off the support you used. Rest in a comfortable position and give yourself time to transition out of this non-ordinary state (*svapna*) of dream-reality.

10. You may wish to draw, write, and read over your captured information. Take some time to reflect on what has come up.

SPANDA® SOMATIC ACCESS TRACKING™ (SPANDA® SAT™)

In this work the body is again attended to in order to elicit information from beneath the waking state. What then comes into awareness can be carefully unraveled to gain insight into the deeper meaning of what is calling to be discovered.

Spanda® Somatic Access Tracking™ developed from my time as a student of Aileen Crow. Aileen was a pioneer in dance-movement therapy and a master somatic therapist who, while a student of Arnold Mindell's Processwork, developed her own perspective on inner body sourcing.

In the late 1970s Arnold Mindell developed a Jungian-based method called Processwork, a part of which connected body experiences with nighttime dreams. He named this non-local field of connection "the dreambody" (Mindell, 2011), in which he found physical symptoms inevitably reflected in dreams and vice versa. He proposed that his notion of the dreambody communicates through body symptoms and experiences, dreams, relationship issues, and world events. While Spanda® Somatic Access Tracking™ is influenced by Crow and Mindell, it is limited to understanding the body's signals in relation to injury and illness. It uses several key concepts from their work. Here we are specifically looking for information that may help navigate a healing potential otherwise overlooked, arising from pain, discomfort, injury or illness. Tying this in with Ballentine's perspective in *Radical Healing* (1999) is the idea that illness or injury may be the symbolic tap on the shoulder from Nature, Beyond, or our higher selves—however you construe this according to your belief system. To me the three are synonymous. The problem may hold information for us that could be the key that helps us evolve toward a more advantageous way of being in the world.

Bringing attention to what is available to perception is an aspect of this work that involves establishing a witness stance. The flow and flux of events available to perception at any moment is the universal expression of *spanda*. The practice of *tapas* is in staying with the signal that has arrived with its irritation, annoyance, hard feeling, or pain. The *tapas* is not only in staying with the signal, it is in inviting and even amplifying the signal by giving it a voice, a chair, and an invitation to "have its say." The dance of *spanda* and *tapas* gives us a window into the information

available to us in the body's signals and symptoms. This only happens if we do not siphon off a signal's energy by allowing it to change channels and dissipate into some activity of relief.

In this somatic practice we track the content signals that arise when paying attention to troubling areas of the body. We work to elicit a signal and then track it as it moves from one channel to another in our awareness. A signal may jump from one channel of awareness to another. For instance, our toe may be tapping the floor outside of our volition or awareness of doing so. But when we bring our attention to the movement, we instantly switch channels and see ourselves running outside in the spring air instead of sitting chained to our desk at work. In this instance we've changed from a kinesthetic to a visual channel. Sometimes a signal change simply reflects the nature of the wandering mind. But, in the case of purposeful attentive focus (*tapasya*), we bring attention to the signal and remain focused on it in its channel. This denies the release of energy and contains its expression. Then we allow other channel attributes to be added to the original signal while not permitting the release of the energy. Doing this provides a fuller expression of the information existing as part of the original signal previously beyond our awareness. At this point we can explore the fullness of the signal and what it may mean in that moment.

It may be that we find ourselves in a memory from long ago, a fantasy scene as if from a fairy tale, or some other reality. If we remain open to what is there, we may decide to investigate some aspect of what has arisen from the dreamscape that is our body's expression. There are many options. We might select a figure and ask what it has to say, or we may embody a dream image and feel its power or gain insight into its perspective. What is important is to stay in touch with what is most interesting and exciting to you. That is the *spandashakti* (authentic creative energy) of the situation and it is how you know what to pursue and what will have meaning.

SOMATIC PRACTICE: Spanda® Somatic Access Tracking™

As above, this practice can be done alone or with a witness-observer.

1. Establish witness consciousness.
2. Allow a signal to arise from the body and note on what channel it arises: visual, proprioceptive, auditory, kinesthetic, or perhaps a combination of these.
3. Boost the signal by focusing your attention on it, adding energy to it. For instance, if you are seeing something, focus on what you are seeing and fill in the details. Or if you are moving, perhaps see if you can make the movement bigger. This is a place in which you are observing yourself, allowing yourself to follow the impulses as they arise, and deciding to enlarge them *while remaining true to their impulse*. One way to tell if you are being true or not is to notice if the work is interesting and exciting. If it feels dead and uninteresting, this often means you've lost the thread of the initial impulse. In this case, simply go back to it and start again.
4. As you boost the signal it will at some point change. It may switch to another channel or add in content from other channels. Just stay with this, continuing to pay attention, and remain true to the impulse as arising from your feeling of yourself in your body. Observe what arises.
5. As this goes on, a more fully formed figure, scene, or event may come into your awareness. Simply continue and observe your responses to it.
6. This next step is optional. You may wish to remain simply observing what has come up or, if you like, you can begin to interact with any of the imagery or figures that have come to the field of your awareness. Think of the content as that of a dream. The items are not real, they are part of the imaginary field your body-mind has conjured into your awareness. So it might be that you turn to ask that stump you just tripped on what it is there for. Of course, in real life the stump won't answer, but in a dream it might. Or you might even become the stump and speak to yourself, saying what comes into awareness as you play this character in your dream. Anything is possible. What is important is to remain connected to your curiosity and what interests you about this. In my experience, curiosity is your Virgil here to lead you through the underworld to what you need to discover.
7. When you come to a point of being able to stop, bring your awareness again to "the ordinary world" of your waking state by paying attention to the space around you. Be aware of the present moment. If you are working with someone, make eye contact.
8. Capture any impressions and if you are working with someone perhaps share your thoughts and impressions.
9. Reflect on the imprints of what you've experienced. How is this about you and your condition, healing challenge, health crisis, or bodily discomfort?

Certainly, at times a symptom is merely that. But, at other times, especially when we find ourselves circling an issue with no apparent way beyond it, it can be useful to entertain that a symptom could hold information for us just outside our awareness. By exploring what occurs when we

SOMATIC *SVADHYAYA* PRACTICE: SELF-INQUIRY WITH THE BODY AS SOURCE   185

pay attention to the information as signals from deeper levels of our being, we may locate parts of ourselves that bring in resources on our quest for healing that have been long forgotten.

Insights you glean from practice may result in changes that propel you along a path of realization of the larger self within. A figure from the pantheon of our individual and collective field of consciousness may bring in something fresh and new. A scene or storyline may recount a universal truth, the mythic form of which we are enduring at this moment in our personal healing journey. Exploring what is there beyond our ego-identity is in service to the evolution of consciousness.

Looking at illness and injury from the point of view of its potential for self-transformation must be done without blame or judgment of the person suffering. Considering symptoms, bodily sensations, and other information usually seen as negative and to be gotten rid of as soon as possible as important sources of insight for healing is contrary to most modern approaches. From a wider perspective, in which the self includes what is beyond the smaller ego-identity, information "stuck" outside and split off from awareness could be trying to make itself known to consciousness. This inclusiveness is a pathway to wholeness. Here symptoms may serve as the seeds of their own medicine. In this larger framework, issues then present themselves in service to the grand goal of the evolution of individual and collective consciousness. This evolution is the main premise of yoga—and its purpose.

Section IV

SOMATIC PRACTICE FOR UNION: YOGA

We are not human beings having a spiritual experience but spiritual beings having a human one.

Georges I. Gurdjieff (in Timms, 1994, p. 62)

INTRODUCTION: THE BODY AS MEDIUM OF ILLUMINATION

Enlightenment is experiential—at least up to the point of union. Experience is how we know where we are on the path. Yoga's original and enduring goal is spiritual development. Its practices were designed primarily to cultivate awareness and discernment. Due to the materialistic nature of modern life and its influence on yoga, yoga today has been taught and practiced with lack of awareness and attention to inner experience. Subtle awareness is a necessary skill for achieving higher states of consciousness. The earlier rungs of yoga are not merely perfunctory, they provide the foundational learning field within which one develops the sensitivities and processes of discrimination needed to attend to the subtler inner cues that act as guideposts in progress on the path.

The body's role in this is very important. The body is itself the ground of our awareness, the home and vehicle of our life processes and experiences. It is the means of our exchange with the world. As such it presents itself as an obstacle requiring attention in maintenance, cleansing, management of "the four fountains" of life: the urges for food, sex, sleep, and self-preservation.

At a more profound level the body is the utensil of our consciousness—the medium of our own sense-making inner reality. As the locale of our neuroreceptive awareness, the body also registers our understanding and is the medium through which we learn and then acknowledge our understanding as a felt sense. As we cultivate our discernment through experience, we note what we experience internally and externally, interpreting our perceptions. We assign meaning and import to them. In this way the body is the basis of our understanding. All these features of our corporality are included in what traditional yoga is designed to address.

THE TRADITIONAL THREADS OF PRACTICE

The traditional yoga lineage from which I teach is an orchestration of three threads. Each thread is entire but here is woven together with other threads to make up a new whole. These threads are sometimes represented as a pyramid, with the lower portions being more accessible and appropriate for larger numbers of people. The first thread and base of the pyramid is Raja Yoga, also known as Ashtanga Yoga. It refers to the eight limbs described by Patanjali in the Yoga Sutras. It is intended as a catholic path of yoga in that it is widely useful for many people.

The second thread is more specialized in that it does not appeal to everyone's character. It is a contemplative path embracing the practice of self-inquiry (*atman vichara*). Advaita Vedanta explores the question "Who am I?" and acknowledges the illusory appearance of the phenomenal world. Practices may include deep reflection (*svadhyaya*) based on the great sayings (*mahavakyas*) of the Upanishads.

The third thread, Samaya Srividya Tantra, addresses an even more particular group of individuals (*adhikars*), and is pictured as the top of the pyramid. Its teachings are shared with those who qualify for this orientation. It may be no surprise that the qualifying features for its advanced practices include a well-developed *buddhi* centered at Ajna Chakra (the third eye), an impeccable ethical compass, and a zeal to reach yoga's final goal. At this point, practices given by an adept are personalized according to the individual's needs. It is important to note that sincere students at every level are taught and become eligible for initiation into this tradition irrespective of gender, religion, race and socioeconomic-ethnic background.

While practicing and developing my work within this profound lineage, one of its senior teachers branched out into specialized work. The work was for those suspecting activation of something holy within. Lacking a context for understanding and working with what is experienced, which is often presenting physical symptoms with no known medical cause, this work filled a special need. The specialized path of Traditional Kundalini Vidya serves people who have what are known as Kundalini risings. In addition to being based in a similar blend of philosophical influences as above, its teachings include knowledge of Kundalini process with the intention of helping individuals progress. Traditional Kundalini Vidya helps someone with a rising understand what is in fact going on and guides them accordingly. Comprehending that a rising is a blessed event rather than a mysterious illness or some sort of madness, an individual can be guided along the path of spiritual development. A spiritual lifestyle with correct guidance can help a Kundalini process progress, which is its goal. As Swami Satchidananda famously said, "Truth is One, Paths are Many" (1978, Ch. 43), and so it is with Kundalini process.

Individualized practices done under the supervision of an adept with careful reporting of experience is an exceptional gift. The subtlety of embodied experiential awareness is crucial in understanding what progress is being made. The subtle work of traditional yoga at advanced stages requires an established stable state of equanimity in the *vijnanamaya kosha*. This is needed so the unloading of latent impressions happens. The *buddhi* (power of discrimination) becomes an even more refined instrument as *sattva* (principle of purity, balance, and light) begins to prevail.

While yoga therapy's emphasis may be on personal wellness, it operates within the framework of yoga. Below I show how yoga practices need not be dissected out of the traditional framework to be effective as a modern wellness modality.

THE *SHATKONA* MODEL: TRADITIONAL YOGA IN THE UPWARD SPIRAL OF YOGA THERAPY

The way in which I place the teachings of my traditions in the context of modern yoga therapy practice came to me as a geometric shape that filled in over time. It became a six-pointed star (*shatkona*). It arose from introspective work I was doing to unload my unconscious and subtle body of deep patterns of perception and reactivity. The star took the form of a three-dimensional spiral with each point of the star at a slightly higher level of ascension. After I drew the star, I recognized I was also illustrating, in my own way, the threads of my traditions as illustrated in pyramidal form (see Figure SIV.1). The pathway from more external focus to more internal work is depicted as well, moving from identity with individual self to that with the universal self. The six areas of remedy from most external to internal are:

1. Knowledge or Education (*vidya*): It is important for clients and students to learn about and understand the framework of yoga, its tenets, and how it works. This helps manage expectations.
2. Lifestyle (*jivacharya*): When giving yoga practices and looking for results it is difficult to expect them if the client's lifestyle is such that it overloads their system regularly or undoes all their fledgling efforts. Lifestyle guidance is important at all levels, but especially at the beginning when results are needed for investment in the practices to continue.
3. Practice (*abhyasa*): These are the classical practices of postures and related *vinyasa* movements, breathing (*pranayama*), relaxation, chanting, meditation, and the like.

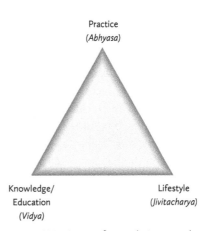

Figure SIV.1 Areas of remedy in yoga therapy for outer *koshic* levels: The triangle

At the next level are the more interior practices (see Figure SIV.2):

4. Self-study and reflection (*svadhyaya*): Self-study is a very important aspect of untangling the thoughts, beliefs, and patterns of our interior world. These patterns may be hidden from view unless explored through somatic practice capable of observing the subtle resultant impulses of energy and thought that impede us from yoga's goal.
5. Faith (*shraddha*): At first, faith as a part of yoga may seem out of place, but it does not need to be in a greater power. It can look simply like hope, or confidence in the process of healing, in the efficacy of yoga, in the relationship with the therapist, or even in the family member who brought the client to the yoga therapy appointment. When we add these two additional aspects, we have a fuller bank of options for deep repatterning and growth.

To complete the image of the whole person there is one more often hidden factor. It is:

6.   Grace (*kripaa*): At times this essential gets omitted for being too spiritual, personal, or unreliable. In therapeutic practice it's useful to recognize that we can't know all the factors at play in illness, restitution, and health. There may be bigger arcs to the storyline out of our view. Conversely, healing as personal transformation can happen when more than what is known is at play. A yogic point of view sees each person not as separate but as part of a larger whole. We are rooted in the Divine.

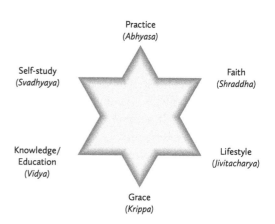

Figure SIV.2 Areas of remedy in yoga therapy: The six-pointed star (*shatkona*)

EXPERIENTIAL AWARENESS AS A TOOL FOR CHANGE

In yoga therapy we may spend the largest portion of our time working with an individual on the maintenance and balance of the physical system. We focus on education about what yoga is, how its practices can help, and how to practice them. We focus on making small sustainable lifestyle changes, while perhaps employing simple Ayurvedic principles like daily routine. We may teach some of yoga's cleansing activities such as nasal wash (*jala neti*). And we give yoga practices like *asana*, relaxation, diaphragmatic breathing, an appropriate version of *agni sara*, and the like. With guided gradual implementation of these foundational, yet often profoundly efficacious methods, we are well equipped to solve the presenting issue.

But there are others who, for one reason or another, are ready for deeper exploration and work. This readiness may even emerge as they purify their body and clarify their mind. It is here that the initial training in experiential awareness becomes the tool for enacting the deep permanent psychological transformation that is next to occur.

On the outside, progress from this deep inner work of self-understanding may look like better self-regulation through the development of functional strategies to deal with the challenges of life while moving out of the cycles that bind. This is enabled through *svadhyaya* and through an ever-deepening understanding of the power and possibility that true yoga provides. Yoga is a path to freedom. As the work is done, that freedom gradually begins to become more apparent to the practitioner.

As it does so, a certain faith begins to occur. It may not necessarily be in God or even something markedly spiritual, but simply in the prospect of improvement. In yoga therapy it may take the form of trust in yoga as a process of betterment, in its philosophy, in its practice. Hope, the item left in Pandora's box when all human ills have been unleashed, is a necessary ingredient in the work of healing. And it, too, is a felt phenomenon.

Beyond the preparation and work on our own part, with proper guidance and sincere, consistent effort, we must at some point also yield to the infinite within and around us. We practice yoga to bolster our physical wellness, emotional and mental stability, and powers of clarity and discernment to put in place the conditions for grace. The reason for surrender is because grace is not something we can ourselves bestow.

What appears next are central practices from the catholic or broad path of Traditional Raja Yoga. What I'll omit here as too wide a subject for this work is the lifestyle guidance for which yoga therapy may call on basic Ayurvedic principles, as well as the *shat kriyas* (six cleansing actions), vegetarianism, and the like. Interestingly, many of these wellness practices have at this time been well integrated into contemporary wellness practice as they are effective and applicable to suffering humanity across the board.

During the 1970s and 1980s a person studying yoga in the United States would likely have been well exposed to these basic yoga practices as they are universal—with some variation—throughout most of the lineages that were brought to the west at that time. These days, as yoga has been deconstructed to fit multifarious objectives, least of which is spiritual advancement, many of these systematic and foundational practices may be widely unknown.

CHAPTER 10

Classical Yoga Practices as a Somatic System of Self-Realization

One time, Swami Rama held a seminar at the Himalayan Institute called The Path of Fire and Light. It was strictly for advanced students. The general mood was that at long last he would impart the secret sacred teachings of the tradition to those of us who'd been diligent in our practice and deserving of next-level practices. The auditorium brimmed with people exuding the natural beauty and confidence that yoga practice imbues, excited to learn the new techniques. But what did he teach? Basic practices—like the ones you'll find below. After the morning session, there was much lunchroom discussion as to what was going on and why this was the case. Was there too much ego in the room? Were people breathing incorrectly? As a creator of mysteries, Swami Rama never explained himself. To this day he has left much about his actions up for interpretation, like a Zen *koan* given to his students to work on and settle in their own hearts. My takeaway was that the most esoteric and transformational experiences are to be found in the most mundane and simplest of practices. This is because it is not the form of the practice that reveals the adeptness of the practitioner, it is the relationship the practitioner has with the form that matters. And this relationship is somatic; it is a felt known reality that is experienced.

This is not to deny that there are more difficult practices to do physically. And mastery of them is quite a feat, albeit a passing one, as everyone's physical body eventually will age—even

yogis'! And this is not to say that a specialized practice designed by an adept cannot speed progress along; this is true in my experience. But it is to say that you can have direct experience of truth without a lot of bells and whistles when you humbly walk the path before you. Below I share with you a host of common basic tools with which you can get there.

Yoga practice is the ultimate somatic practice when done with awareness. In its various physical practices we learn how to examine our "tissues for issues" of weakness or lack of vitality and remedy them with position and breath and movement. On a deeper, more integral level, we can use the interface of body, energy, and felt sense to examine our programmable responses to life. And, on the mental level, in which the body is stilled for work with the mind, we are then able to apply the same principles of awareness, differentiation, and understanding to sort through our habits, thoughts, emotions, and actions. Through the practice of authentic yoga we are able to understand our deeply personal hang-ups and issues and work toward their remedy.

As yoga therapists we turn these very same self-reflective skills outward to observe others. The International Association of Yoga Therapists' standards for the practice of yoga therapy require practitioners to layer other frameworks over yoga, those of allopathic medicine, anatomy, and mental health perspectives. But the basis of the practice remains yoga; and yoga is an embodied path of deliverance to grace.

What follows is a compilation of what I consider central basic practices selected from Raja Yoga. Here I'll give the common version. Each practice can be adapted and modified according to need from these aspects of practice: *yama* and *niyama*, *asana*, *pranayama*, relaxation and meditation. The order below roughly follows the progression of the eight limbs of Ashtanga: *yama*, *niyama*, *asana*, *pranayama*, *pratyahara*, *dharana*, *dhyana*, and *samadhi*, although there is great variety possible in implementing each of these in practice. And that is perhaps precisely one reason why yoga therapy is such a salient and effective method of care; it can serve as a great reservoir of principles and practices that are systematic and effective. When applied judiciously and with attentive care, the practices work in harmony with the laws of nature and benefit us optimally. We'll begin with the first two rungs.

PURIFICATION, OR ADDING TO THE DILEMMA: *YAMA* AND *NIYAMA*

Of Patanjali's eight-limbed path, the first two limbs, *yama* and *niyama*, offer guidance in how to basically stay out of trouble in life. When you think about it, all actions have results, and those results are either helpful or not on the path to union. You must do actions in life. The question, then, is how to make the actions you do as harmless as possible. A sincere yoga practitioner will practice yoga throughout every minute of their life, not just on their yoga mat.

The five *yama* are also called the five restraints. Their purpose is to help us temper our more primitive reptilian nature. Keeping these directives in play helps us manage our desires and in so doing fosters healthy relationships. They are: non-harming (*ahimsa*), truthfulness (*satya*), non-stealing (*asteya*), moderation of the senses (*brahmacharya*), and non-possessiveness (*aparigraha*). Practicing these as attitudes help us regulate the disturbances of body and mind created by the senses and the four primitive urges (sleep, sex, hunger, self-preservation.) As somatic practice, adherence to the *yama* gives us a stress-reduced embodiment. Through the moral code they provide we lessen our negative impact and need for protection. Our lives become simpler and the lack of need for duplicity of character can be felt in the body and experienced as a deepening of ease.

The five *niyama* are also called the observances. They help us focus our innate drive (*spanda*) toward the goal of yoga by inspiring and supporting us in remaining in touch with our own self-guidance within. They are purity (*saucha*), contentment (*santosha*), self-discipline (*tapas*), scriptural and self-study (*svadhyaya*), and surrender to the highest good (*ishvara pranidhana*). As our lives center more consistently around the source of our being, we experience a lightness and consistency that can felt as *sattva* in the body-mind. Both the *yama* and *niyama* provide us with tools for maintaining and recovering balance in life, resulting in a lessening of dysregulation of our nervous system.

SOMATIC PRACTICE: *Yama* and *niyama*

I have always thought of the *yama* and *niyama* as path-clearers. When a sincere student of yoga practices steadfastly, things begin to change within them. Behavior is complex. So the self-study centered on these guiding principles will not necessarily show up directly as an instant result—although at times it might. The practice is one of introspection centered on how you feel yourself to be, or, in the words of contemporary discourse, on your neuroceptive awareness. This is what you notice when you read your body. How do you feel? How is your stress level? Are your muscles tight, is your digestion great or off, can your mind hold its focus well? These and all other manner of check-ins can reveal how close to or far from a *sattvic* state of clarity and ease, with the possibility of delight, you are. If these are good, it's a sign that these principles are operating well in your life!

1. Choose one of the *yama* or *niyama* as your focus and set the amount of time you'll spend practicing this principle in all your affairs: a day or two or a week is a good start.
   a. Non-harming (*ahimsa*)
   b. Truthfulness (*satya*)
   c. Non-stealing (*asteya*)
   d. Moderation of the senses (*brahmacharya*)
   e. Non-possessiveness (*aparigraha*)
   f. Purity (*saucha*)
   g. Contentment (*santosha*)
   h. Self-discipline (*tapas*)
   i. Scriptural and self-study (*svadhyaya*)
   j. Surrender to the highest good (*ishvara pranidhana*).
2. As you go through your day, notice any behavior that involves this principle primarily in yourself but also in the people you encounter live and over the media. Perhaps you've chosen truthfulness or *satya*. Notice the interactions you have in which this behavior is relevant, in your work, in your family life, in your own self-talk.
3. Then find a time later in the day for playback of encounters. Notice any in which there may have been an issue with honesty, especially if you've noticed a gray area, in which perhaps not telling the truth would save you embarrassment at work or just save time. No matter what behavior you did, replay the event with *satya* not at play, and then again with it in place. As you do this, track your felt response. Notice how your body feels.

For instance, when I replay an incident in which it was easier to just not share the truth to save time, even though the matter took less time, I notice a sinking feeling in my chest under my breastbone and that my inhale is not as full as before this replay. When I replay with honesty, this feeling, that I now associate with shame and hiding, does not arise in my body. Instead I feel my breath ground deeper in my rib cage as my ribs flare slightly to the sides. I associate this felt sense with patience and uprightness. I am ready for a reaction and in a good place from which to negotiate.

I believe our bodies cannot lie. We'll have a response, possibly a very subtle one at times, to our thoughts, feelings, and actions that can help us navigate our way in the world. These principles intersect and overlap. For instance, I might decide not to share the truth in a situation where I deem it would prove harmful to someone. I mitigate my responses in an effort to enact the highest good. My body's responses act as my compass for such decisions. As I strive to make good ones I can live with, yoga instructs me to use my body as the messenger as to whether or not that is truly so.

POINTS OF DEPARTURE: *ASANA* (POSTURES)

A balanced classical *asana* practice, as I call it, will bring the body's energy into harmony, balance the physiological tone of the various tissues and autonomic system, and work to eliminate blockages and impediments of flow. It will also bring life energy to the main vertical lines of energy movement in the body, along several pathways called the *shakti nadis*. These are like interstate highways for energy to travel upward physically and metaphysically in our experience of ourselves at all levels of our being. A regular, reasonable, balanced practice clears the roads, so to speak, and makes the way ready for the bestowing of grace.

At one point I researched the presentation of *asana* across various traditions. I was curious about how a practitioner progressed from one element of a practice routine to another in that session, and what types or categories of *asana*, such as back bends or twists, we standardly included. I was taught a progression from standing to sitting to lying down with inversion as the final practice just prior to relaxation. *Pranayama* as an isolated practice (not in combination with *asana* or *vinyasa*) could be inserted at the beginning, between standing and floor work, and at the end. My research yielded a conglomerate of what I considered a complete classical practice that hit all the main categories.

A balanced classical practice will then include at least one practice per category. Some poses, however, fall into more than one practice category. A great range of ability can be achieved within this formula as it can be altered as needed and still be full and well balanced. Also, *vinyasa* sequences may move through several poses in various ways.

SOMATIC PRACTICE: A balanced classical practice

This work assumes some knowledge of yoga practice. In all cases, please use these directions as a guide for your practice and feel free to change them as you see fit by paying attention to your body and its sensations. The somatic practice here is to learn the practices and perform them to your comfortable capacity. Pay attention to your experience as you do. Listen to your body and your mind. If you are inclined to explore in this way over time, examine your sense of well-being, overall energy, and emotional state. What do you notice?

Relaxation and breathing practice

'You may want to start with a centering practice such as relaxation and breathing.'

Joint and general limbering

To gently warm up, complete some repetitive circling movements at the major joints of wrists, shoulders, hips, and ankles. Fold forward with knees slightly bent and come up a few times gently while breathing fully. Lift the knees, marching in place. Swing arms and twist easily side to side. Do any other gentle limbering movements you like.

Heating movement and *vinyasa*
Sun Salutation (*Surya Namaskar*)
(Figures 10.1–10.11)

1. Stand tall in Mountain Pose (*Tadasana*); exhale.
2. Inhale and raise the arms overhead, forearms near the ears. Exhale and stretch upward.

3. Inhale and arch up and back, slightly bending the knees and allowing the pelvis to move slightly forward (*Urdhvasana*). Exhale here.

4. Inhale and extend upward to stand again with arms overhead.

5. Exhale while reaching forward, bending at the hips. Aim the top of the head toward the floor as you can and let the arms fall.

6. Inhale and step your right foot back into a lunge position. Inhale here.

7. Exhale and step the other foot back while lowering the body to the floor like this: drop your knees, chest, and nose toward the floor (*Ashtanamaskarasana*). Then allow the rest of the body onto the floor.

8. Inhale and lead with your nose to lift upward into a low arched position, keeping the elbows bent and palms on the floor.

9. Exhale and lower down.

10. Inhale, tuck your toes, and get ready to push.

11. Exhale. Push with your hands, bend at the hips, and reach the pelvis up and back on a diagonal into Downward-facing Dog Pose (*Adho Mukha Shvanasana*).

12. If you like, you can now bring both knees to the floor as an intermediary position or go right from Down Dog. Then inhale and bring the right foot forward between the hands to a lunge.

13. Exhale and push from the back toes to step the feet next to one another. You should be in some form of a forward fold pose (*Uttanasana*).

14. Inhale and hinge upward to stand with the arms overhead; do this in a way that suits your back!

15. Exhale while bringing your arms down to your sides.

16. Repeat with the other foot leading.

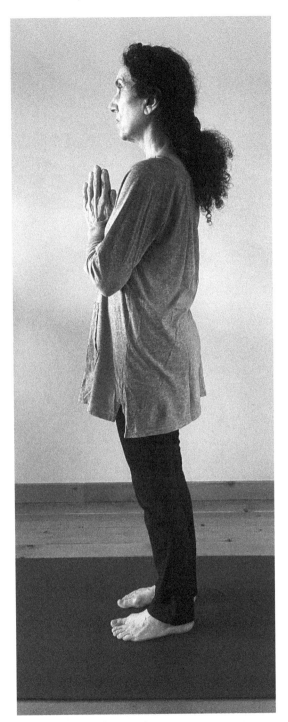

Figure 10.1 Sun Salutation A

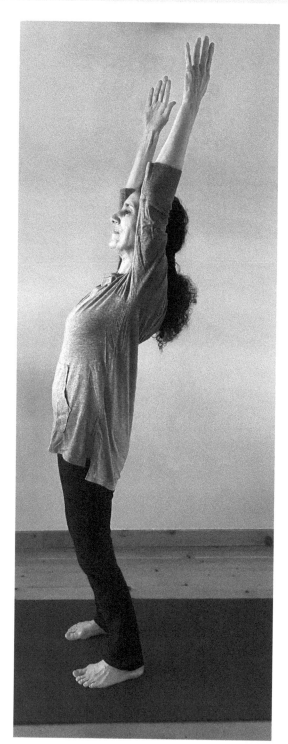

Figure 10.2 Sun Salutation B

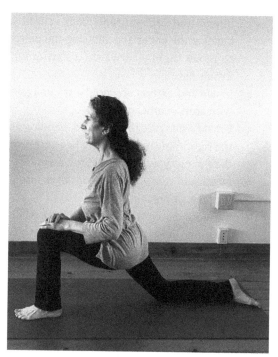

Figure 10.3 Sun Salutation C

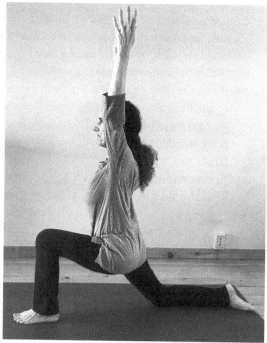

Figure 10.4 Sun Salutation D

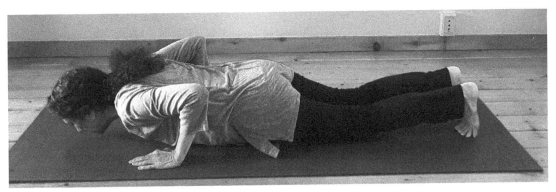

Figure 10.5 Sun Salutation E

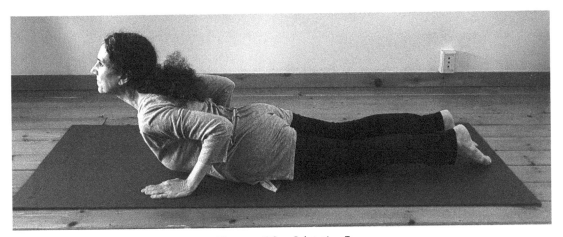

Figure 10.6 Sun Salutation F

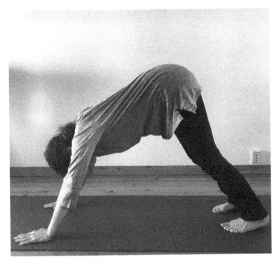

Figure 10.7 Sun Salutation G

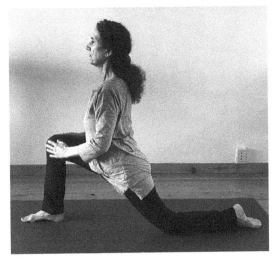

Figure 10.8 Sun Salutation H

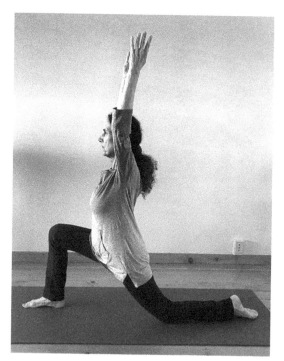

Figure 10.9 Sun Salutation I

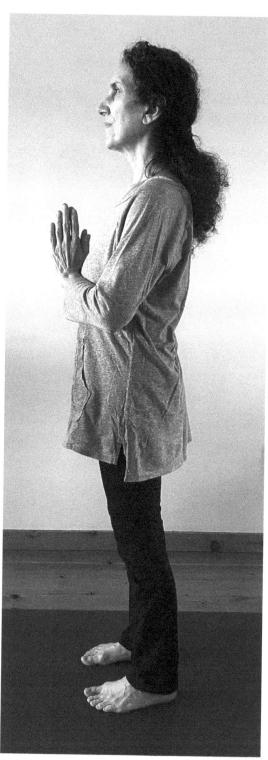

Figure 10.11 Sun Salutation K

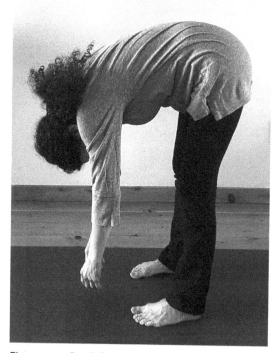

Figure 10.10 Sun Salutation J

Pelvic centering (*Agni Sara Dhouti*) (*Figure 10.12*)

In this practice you coordinate the contractions of your pelvic floor and abdominal wall, which may take some getting used to.

1. Stand with feet slightly wider than your hips. Tilt forward from your hips, keeping your back straight, and place your hands on your thighs.
2. As you exhale, draw upward from the pelvic floor to your stomach.
3. As you inhale, release the contraction sequentially from top to bottom.
4. Repeat several times. You can work up to 25 times once you have mastered the movement.

This exercise has some important precautions. Please do not do this when pregnant, or if you have colitis, intestinal ulcer, hiatal hernia, unmedicated high blood pressure, glaucoma, raised intracranial pressure, or overactive thyroid.

Whole body integration in the Extended Triangle Pose (*Utthita Trikonasana*) (*Figure 10.13*)

1. Stand with legs apart. Rotate your left leg outward 90 degrees and your right leg inward 45 degrees.
2. Inhale, stretch your arms out to the sides at shoulder height, palms facing forward.
3. Exhale, bend to the left from your hips, keeping your body flat to the side. Place your left hand on your shin, foot, or the floor according to your comfortable capacity.
4. Keep the right arm high above your right shoulder, looking forward. Breathe evenly and remain in the pose for several breaths.
5. Press your left heel into the floor as you bring your torso back to standing wide. Step together.
6. Repeat the practice on the other side.

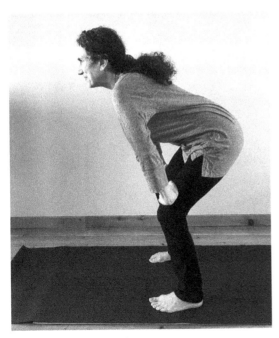

Figure 10.12 *Agni Sara Dhouti*

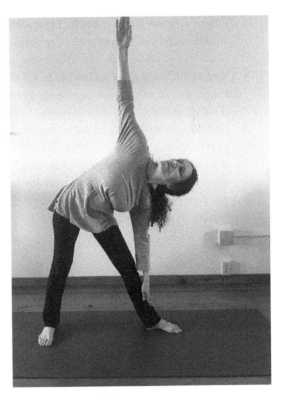

Figure 10.13 Triangle Pose

A favorite standing posture: Warrior Pose (*Virabhadrasana*)

1. Stand with legs wide apart. Rotate your left leg outward 90 degrees and your right leg inward 45 degrees. Turn your pelvis so that it faces diagonally to the left.
2. Inhale, elongate your spine as you raise the arms overhead, palms facing one another.
3. Breathe fully, noticing the alignment of your feet, legs, and torso. Release your effort as you breathe deep, even, and full. Stay to your comfortable capacity.
4. To come out of the pose, pivot your back leg to a parallel position then push off to step together facing the side. Repeat on the other side.

Balance in Tree Pose (*Vrikshasana*) (Figure 10.14)

1. Stand with legs together.
2. Rotate your left leg to the side, bend your left knee, and place your foot on the inside of your right ankle, shin, or at the knee.
3. Inhale and bring your palms together at your chest or raise them overhead, keep the back straight.
4. Breathe evenly as you balance, focusing your gaze on one spot in front of you. Stay to your comfortable capacity. Then slowly allow the arms and raised leg to return to standing position.
5. Repeat on the other side.

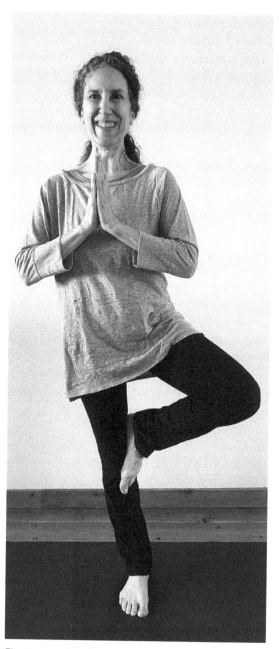

Figure 10.14 Tree Pose

Side bending in Standing Half Moon Side Bend Pose (*Ardha Chandrasana*) (Figure 10.15)

1. Stand with your feet hip-width apart. Inhale and raise your right arm overhead.
2. Exhale while reaching up and over to the left, bending to your left side from your waist. Try to remain flat to the side, not allowing your body to round forward. Hold and breathe. Stay to your comfortable capacity.
3. Inhale to return to upright.
4. Exhale, lower the right arm.
5. Repeat on the other side. You may also wish to try this with both arms raised.

A pranayama practice could be inserted here.

Backward bending in Cobra Pose (*Bhujangasana*) (Figure 10.16)

Please do not perform this pose if you have stomach or duodenal ulcer, a hernia, or hyperthyroidism.

1. Lie on the floor prone, with palms on the floor next to your chest.
2. Exhale and reach your mouth forward so you feel a gentle stretch in the throat area.
3. Inhale and slowly peel your body off the floor one vertebra at a time, leading up and back with the top of your head. Use your back muscles and not your arms, which are there for stability, not weight bearing.
4. Hold while breathing optimally for as long as you like.
5. Slowly return your torso to the floor and then your head, turning it to either side. Bring the arms to your sides and notice the effect of the pose.

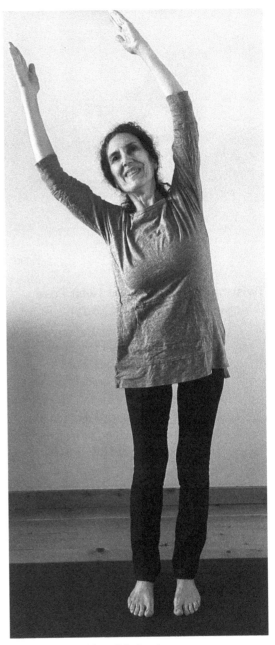

Figure 10.15 Standing Side Bend

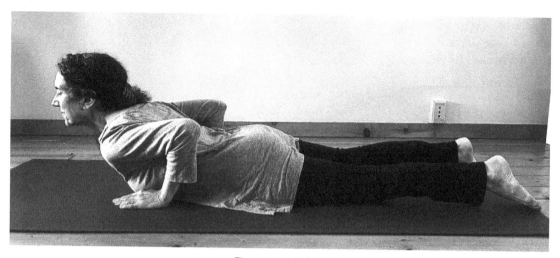

Figure 10.16 Cobra

Twisting in Seated Spinal Twist Pose (*Matsyendrasana*) (Figure 10.17)

1. Sit tall with your legs extended in front. Bend your left knee and place your left foot on the floor at the outside of your right knee, or as close to this as is comfortable. Keep the right leg extended or shift your weight to the right, turning out your right thigh, then bend the right knee and slide the heel toward your left hip.

2. Inhale and press downward through your sitting bones to elongate your spine as you raise your arms overhead.

3. Exhale and twist to the left, lowering your arms. Place your left hand on the floor behind your left hip and turn your head to the back.

4. Hold the pose to your comfortable capacity.

5. To release, inhale to raise the arms overhead while turning your torso and head to the front.

6. Exhale, bringing the arms down and extending the bent leg.

7. Repeat on the other side.

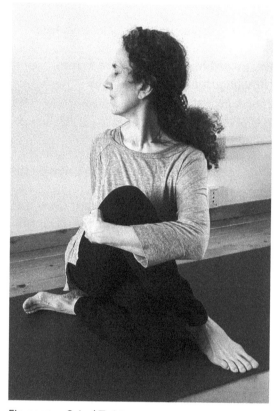

Figure 10.17 Spinal Twist

Forward bending in Posterior Stretch Pose (*Paschimottanasana*) (Figure 10.18)

1. Sit with your legs extended to the front.
2. Inhale and raise your arms overhead, extending your spine upward.
3. Exhale and bend forward from your hips, reaching forward over your legs.
4. Allow your hands to fall onto your legs and gently grasp them, or rest your hands there.
5. Breathe and hold the position, allowing the weight of your head to lengthen your back muscles as much as possible. Hold there to your comfortable capacity.
6. To come out, inhale and reach your head and arms again upward, or allow the arms to fall to the sides of your body, while returning to sitting.

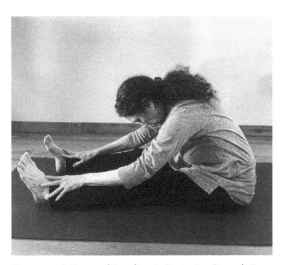

Figure 10.18 Forward Bending in Posterior Stretch Pose

Hip mobility through Bound Angle Pose (*Baddha Konasana*) (Figure 10.19)

1. Sit with the soles of your feet together, knees rotated out to the sides.
2. Inhale and reach the arms overhead, elongating the torso and sitting as tall as you can without strain.
3. Exhale and bend forward from your hips, bringing your arms to the floor in front of you. Breathe and let the head go as far as possible. Remain here as long as you like. If being forward in this position is difficult, simply sit and place the fingertips behind your hips to hold the position to your comfortable capacity.
4. When you are ready to come out of the pose, gently roll up or reach forward again with your head, and inhale as you come back to an upright position.

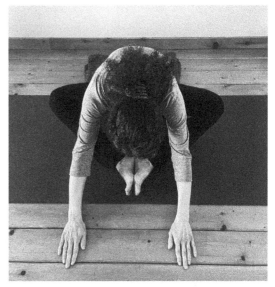

Figure 10.19 Bound Angle

Inversion through Inverted Action Pose (*Viparita Karani*) (Figure 10.20)

Please do not include this pose if you have neck issues.

1. Lie supine with arms next to the body.
2. Exhale, bending the knees and drawing the thighs into your torso.
3. Inhale while extending the legs upward.
4. Exhale, push with your arms, and roll your pelvis off the floor, your legs going over your upper torso and head as possible.
5. Continue breathing evenly as you bend at the elbows to place your hands under your hips for support. You should feel some

of the weight of your lower body travel through your forearms here.

6. Stay to your comfortable capacity.

7. To come out of the pose, release the arms to the floor and, using your abdominal muscles, slowly roll down so your pelvis is again on the floor.

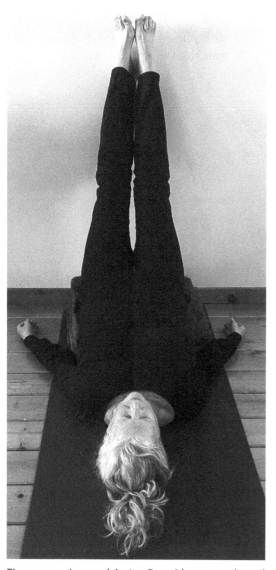

Figure 10.20 Inverted Action Pose (shows an adapted version using a support under the hips and the legs resting on a wall)

Expanding and extending life: *Pranayama*

These practices can be done at the same time as posture practice or at a separate time. When done as part of an *asana* practice session, they may be done at the beginning, at the transition from standing to the floor, or at the end prior to relaxation. This helps one to identify the effects of each practice.

Pranayama refers to the control and expansion of life energy. It is practiced primarily by working with the breath. The breath can be used to relax, steady, and balance the nervous system, improve concentration, and expand and improve the flow of energy in and around the body. As the power grid of our body, working with prana through our breath yields the experience of even, good flow and consistent available energy. Our emotional regulation is also benefited by consistent appropriate regular practice.

Two central practices are described below. The somatic exploration of these, as above, is in the experience of the practice. With *pranayama* is it especially helpful to do a somatic check-in of how you feel overall, energetically if that is something you can track, and emotionally, before and after the practice.

Optimal diaphragmatic breathing

The diaphragm is a dome-shaped muscle located at the bottom of the rib cage. It runs horizontally, attaching down the front of the spine at the lower back. When you breathe in, this dome flattens down like a platter. When you breathe out it relaxes and domes back up to its resting position.

Although diaphragmatic breathing is simple, easy, and beneficial, the habit of doing it often has to be consciously cultivated before it becomes automatic. A simple practice of diaphragmatic breathing is best done at first while lying supine. Optimizing this action of the diaphragm by allowing the breath to be deep and smooth and even without pause will give you the best overall results.

1. Lie on your back on a mat or rug. If you like you can place a small pillow under your head. Place one hand on your stomach just below the bottom of your breastbone. As you breathe in, this area should move upward toward the ceiling; as you breathe out this area should gently fall back toward your spine and the floor. Take your other hand and place it on the chest just above your heart. See if this area is moving more, or less, than the stomach area. It may move a little but, if it is moving more, then see if you can move the breath more from the diaphragm.

2. Now place the hand that was on the chest on your lower abdomen and observe the amount of movement. This area may move a little but, if it is moving more, direct your awareness to the stomach area and move the breath from there. Now allow the arms to rest on the floor, palms facing upward.

3. If possible, breathe only through your nose. Inhale, allow the lower edge of the rib cage to expand slightly as the abdomen rises. As you exhale, allow the abdomen to fall toward the floor and the bottom of the ribs to gently narrow. For the duration of your breath cycle there should be relatively little movement of the upper chest.

4. Next, check on the rate of your breath. Breathing between 16 and 20 breaths per minute is considered average, but slower diaphragmatic breathing is calming and improves oxygen and carbon dioxide exchange in the lungs. Feel inside your torso as your diaphragm descends and displaces the contents of your abdomen forward as you breathe in.

5. Feel the breath in the nostrils, cooler as it comes in, warmed by the body as it goes out. Make this flow of breath even by moving the diaphragm steadily without pause. Notice the ends of the breath cycle: the end of the exhale, the end of the inhale. See if you can smooth out the transitions so that the breath is continuous without pause at either "end."

6. Also, if possible, there should be no sound in the breath. Features of optimal breathing are that the breath flows silently, smoothly, without stops or jerks and there is no pause. This may take some practice.

A ten-minute practice of optimal diaphragmatic breathing is a good start!

If for some reason you cannot start practicing diaphragmatic breathing lying on your back, then try it in Crocodile Pose (*Makarasana*) (Figure 10.21). Lie on the stomach, placing the legs a comfortable distance apart and pointing the toes outward. Fold the arms in front of the body, resting the hands near the opposite elbows. Position the arms so the upper chest does not touch the floor and rest the forehead on the arms.

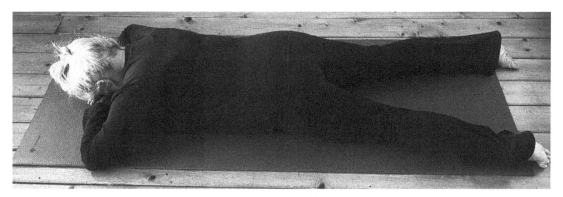

Figure 10.21 Crocodile Pose

This posture allows you to feel the abdomen pressing against the floor as you breathe in, and the abdominal muscles relaxing as you breathe out.

If you find diaphragmatic breathing difficult or confusing (or both!) Sandbag Breathing may help. I'm including this variation here because diaphragmatic breathing is the bedrock of yoga practice in this approach. All else is built on it. Sandbag Breathing strengthens the abdominal muscles and the diaphragm and helps regulate the motion of the lungs in cooperation with the movement of the diaphragm.

Sandbag Breathing (Figure 10.22)

1. Lie on your back in *Shavasana*, and take a moment to relax your body. Now gently place a sandbag of about five pounds or roughly 2.5 kg on your abdomen. If you have a heart, lung, or blood pressure issue or abnormality, place the sandbag lower down near your navel, positioning it so the pelvic bones are not holding most of its weight.
2. Close your eyes and breathe. Feel the sandbag rise as you inhale and drop as you exhale. See if you can center your effort on the muscles that move the bag and nowhere else.
3. After 3–5 minutes remove the sandbag and relax on your back for a few more minutes.

If you practice this regularly you may wish to gradually increase the weight of the sandbag. But do not exceed 15 pounds or 7 kg.

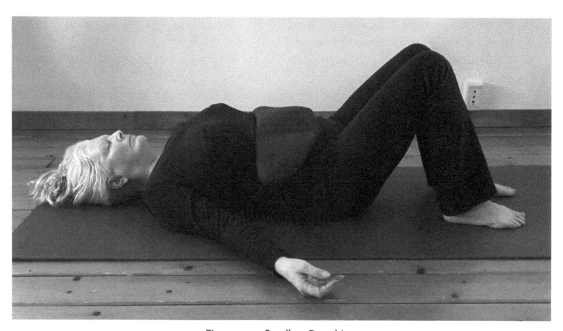

Figure 10.22 Sandbag Breathing

Alternate Nostril Breathing (*Nadi Shodhanam*)

This practice is known to purify the body's energy grid or channels (*nadis*) by slowly and gently alternating the breath flow from one nostril to the other. Of the many versions, this version uses the hands to alternate the breath by gently closing one nostril at a time with no retention of the breath. If for any reason you do not wish to occlude the breath, either due to heart or breathing issues or that you simply don't feel you want to, you can do the practice without the hands. Just visualize the air flow on one side and then the other.

1. Find a stable erect position and breathe diaphragmatically, with a smooth, steady, even, easy rhythm.
2. Determine which nostril is freer by closing one nostril and blowing air out the other nostril alternately. You'll begin by exhaling through the freer nostril.
3. If using your hand, you'll place the thumb of your right hand over your right nostril and the ring finger over the left one. The other fingers can be folded in.
4. Begin by exhaling through the freer nostril.
5. Once you've exhaled through the freer nostril, close it and inhale through the less free nostril. This is one breath cycle. Repeat this twice more.
6. Now begin by exhaling through the more clogged nostril and inhaling through the freer one. Repeat this twice more. You've now done six cycles.
7. Continue with the pattern of three cycles, beginning on one side and then the other for as long as you wish. Five minutes would be a good starting practice.

Once completed, notice the effect. How do you feel? Does the breath flow more evenly between the nostrils? When it does, that is called *sandhya* or "joyous mind." It is a very good set-up for meditation practice.

THE ULTIMATE SOMATIC CHECK-IN: SYSTEMATIC RELAXATION

Relaxation gives rest to the body, especially to any areas of chronic tension, rest to the nervous system, and rest to the mind. Systematic relaxation practice is a practice in which the mind travels through the body and invites each area to release or yield its weight into gravity. As a somatic practice it is unparalleled when done regularly over time. It can count as the ultimate check-in and gives an intimacy of present awareness to and with each and every cell of the body. In Ayurveda there is a term *Khavaigunya*, which refers to a weaker "space" or area or tissue of the body with the tendency toward impairment. As an entire living system we embody our physicality with energy and consciousness/conscious awareness. Bringing conscious awareness to each body part, area, and region, and even in our imagination to each cell as it conducts its activities, is a way to inhabit and take possession of the spaces of our bodily being. Relaxation practice does not only bring our awareness systematically to each and every body area, it instructs us to release any holding, and buildup of waste, and any unnecessary alarm in our tissues. As we move throughout the body in an organized and systematic way, we support the flow of energy that allows our body systems to do their jobs without our mental and emotional interference.

Relaxation practice can be done on its own, in conjunction with meditation, and as a part of any yoga *asana* practice session. Typically, it is done at both the beginning and ending of the practice session, but if there is less time, it is done at the end only. A typical relaxation practice lasts about 8–12 minutes. An abbreviated relaxation can also be interspersed anytime within an *asana* practice between postures. If time is available for this, it is an excellent way to note and integrate the effects of each pose.

These four poses are excellent to use for relaxation practice. *Shavasana* means Corpse Pose, and while this name is a bit macabre it indicates that the body can become extremely still. The state of deep relaxation is a rejuvenative one, so the position that evokes the most ease and stillness is the right one for your practice.

Relaxation postures

Corpse Pose (*Shavasana*): Lie supine, palms up, legs comfortably apart. You may place a folded blanket under your head or neck and under your knees if needed for comfort.

Crocodile Pose (*Makarasana*), described above, can be done with the forehead centered on the back of the hands or wrists, or the head can be turned to one side for greater comfort if needed.

Flapping Fish Pose (*Matsya Kridasana*) (Figure 10.23): Lie prone, turning the head to the right. Bring one knee up along that side and bend the right arm so you are partially on your side and partially on your front. Bring the opposite arm overhead along the floor or bend both elbows and tuck your hands under the side of your head, like a small pillow. Change to the other side as you like.

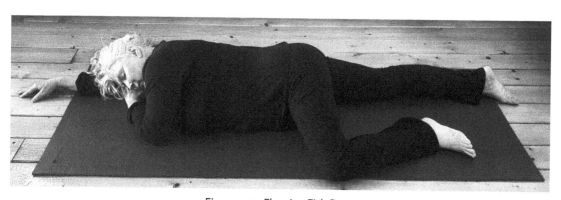

Figure 10.23 Flapping Fish Pose

Friendship Pose (*Maitriasana*) is simply sitting on a chair or bench with head, neck, and trunk aligned, feet flat on the floor.

Head-to-toe systematic relaxation

1. Lie supine in *Shavasana*. You may wish to have a small pillow under your head.
2. Feel the breath in the nostrils, cooler as it comes in, warmed by the body as it goes out. Make this flow of breath even by moving the diaphragm steadily without pause. Notice the ends of the breath cycle: the end of the exhale, and the end of the inhale. See if you can smooth out the transitions so that the breath is continuous without pause at either end.
3. Bring awareness to your head. Allow the weight of the head to relax into the floor. Relax the muscles of your face, flatten the forehead, allow the eyes to fall back into the head, relax the cheeks, allow the jaw to hang, relax the lips. Allow the tongue to relax back into the throat.
4. Relax the neck, allowing the neck muscles to soften and widen. Allow the passageways in the neck to release. Relax the "roots" of the neck muscles that spread into the upper torso. Relax out to the shoulders.
5. Allow the weight of the upper body to release into the floor through the shoulder blades. Travel through the arms and relax the arms. Relax the palms of the heads and the fingers. Relax the fingertips.
6. Relax the entire upper torso from

the neck to the waist. Allow the back muscles to relax. Relax the heart and lungs, and whatever you notice is not fully releasing its weight into the floor in the upper torso area.

7. Relax the waist and the low back area. Feel the weight of the body to release into the floor.

8. Relax the pelvis, the pelvic floor, and the hips. Allow the bowl of the pelvis to rest against the floor and relax the contents of the pelvis back into it.

9. Travel down through the legs with your awareness. Relax the thigh, knees, lower legs. Relax the ankles, feet, and toes. Relax the tips of the toes.

10. Return to the feeling of breathing. Allow the breath to move in a slow even steady circle. Feel the effect of this practice.

When you are ready to come out of this practice, move peripherally, first the hands and feet, wrists and ankles. Gradually move more in any way you like. Then bend your knees and roll to one side. Rest there until you feel ready to sit up.

Relaxation is a skill like others that can be acquired through practice. The more regularly and frequently it is practiced, the more quickly the skill of relaxation is learned.

PREPARING FOR LIFT-OFF: MEDITATION

Meditation allows us to concentrate in a relaxed way so that the mind is able to easily flow toward its object. The practice helps us develop our inner witness or the part of us able to remain relatively objective. As the mind becomes quiet, it is possible to study its content with increasing clarity and discernment.

These five steps are the preparation for the experience of meditation. All of the yoga practices work together to optimize the conditions for successful meditation, and these five items when done in succession directly support a meditative state. It's like the other aspects of Ashtanga are the vehicles in which we arrive at the castle gate. The five steps below open the gate and take us to the entrance door, upon which we knock with the repetition of our mantra. The rest is Grace.

This practice uses the mental repetition of a sound or mantra. A mantra that supports optimal breathing, and can be done by everyone, is *soham*. The sound "so" is recited on inhalation, "ham" on exhalation. The sounds are not spoken out loud but repeated mentally. Soham mimics to some degree the natural sound of breathing, and is translated as "I am That," with "That" being one's Divine nature, or "I am who I am."

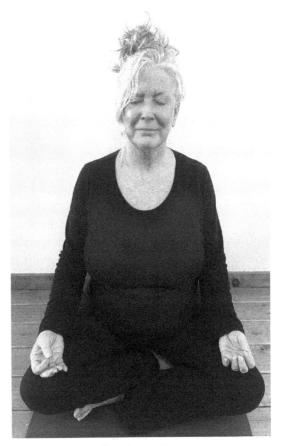

Figure 10.24 Seated Meditation Pose

Five-Step Meditation preparation

1. *Physical stillness*: Choose a seated posture in which the head, neck, and trunk can be aligned (Figure 10.24). You may wish to explore various sitting postures, then choose one that's comfortable and that you can remain in for a period of time.
2. *Rhythmic diaphragmatic breathing*: Bring your attention to the feeling of breathing. Feel the flow of breath through the nostrils—cooler on the inhale, warmer on the exhale. Feel the diaphragm muscle descend and flatten like a large platter on the inhale, and dome back up under the bottom of the rib cage on the exhale. Allow the breath to be even, smooth, and steady, without pause.
3. *Systematic relaxation*: While maintaining physical stillness and rhythmic diaphragmatic breathing, systematically relax each area of the body from head to toe. Relax what you notice is unnecessarily active while remaining seated.
4. *Breath awareness*: Allow the mind to rest on the steady movement of the breath. This begins the formal practice. If the mind strays from this task, simply bring it back without comment or further disruption. You may also practice Alternate Nostril Breathing here.
5. *Mantra repetition*: A mantra is a sound or series of sounds used as the object of focus. Use gentle effort to keep your mind focused on mentally repeating the sound. As above, as the mind wanders, gently bring it back to this task. Over time the sound repetition will become more automatic and spontaneous.

The best times for meditation practice are before breakfast, lunch, and dinner, and prior to sleep if it does not keep you from falling asleep. As the ability to witness develops, meditation allows us better stability for self-study of habit patterns and unconscious impediments to wellness and growth. As we unload our karma, we become clearer, lighter, and more stable in the awareness of who we truly are.

A COMPLETE PRACTICE

While this is merely a beginning glimpse of the practice, it is a good starting somatic series of practices to give a sense of the effects of the practices on your state of being. Yoga is a systematic science of self-realization in which no effort is ever wasted.

For a more pointed experience of how the somatic practices of yoga lead to a state of purification, equilibrium, a deep state of peace, and perhaps even beyond, the practice below is included. It attends to the body's energy grid or sheath, the *prana maya kosha*, centering attention on several of its confluences or centers. Visualization and mental repetition of sound are also used in conjunction with the traveling of awareness through the body. As in all the practices, it remains important to observe your state of being before, during, and after the practice to fully experience its benefit.

Purification of the elements: *Bhuta Shuddhi* (ascending breath variation)
If you are experiencing mental illness of any sort, please omit this practice at this time.

1. Close your eyes and focus your attention at the base of your spine. This is the Muladhara Chakra, the abode of the earth element. Here visualize a yellow square surrounded by four petals.

Mentally repeat "*lam*," the *bija* (seed) mantra of the earth element, 16 times, while focusing at the Muladhara.

2. Next, focus your attention just above the root of the genitals or at the uterus. Visualize the Svadhishthana Chakra, the abode of the water element, as an ocean-blue circle with a white crescent moon in the center. The circle is surrounded by six petals. While you maintain this image, mentally repeat the *bija* mantra of the water element, "*vam*," 16 times.

3. Now focus your awareness at your navel center. Visualize the Manipura Chakra, the abode of fire here, a red triangle pointing upward. This triangle is enclosed in a circle of ten petals. Mentally repeat the *bija* mantra of the fire element, "*ram*," 16 times.

4. Next focus your awareness at your heart center and visualize the *anahata*, which is the abode of air, as two smoky-gray triangles, one superimposed upon the other, encircled by a 12-petaled lotus. At this stage mentally repeat the *bija* mantra of the air element, "*yam*," 16 times.

5. Next focus your awareness at the base of your throat. Visualize the Vishuddha Chakra, the abode of ether, as a sky-blue circle surrounded by a 16-petaled lotus. The presiding force of this chakra is contained in the *bija* mantra of the space (or ether) element, *ham*. Repeat 16 times.

6. Now focus your awareness between and a little above your eyebrows. Visualize the Ajna Chakra, the realm of mind, as a yellow triangle surrounded by a circle. A bright white flame is enclosed in the triangle. Outside the circle are two petals. Mentally repeat the mantra "*so hum*" or "*Om*" 16 times.

7. Now bring awareness to the top of your head. This is the realm of the Sahasrara Chakra, the thousand-petaled crown center which is the abode of pure consciousness. At this center all colors, forms, and shapes dissolve as this chakra is beyond the mind and therefore beyond imagination. It can be experienced as countless rays of white light. However, it is often visualized as a thousand-petaled lotus with a pinkish aura so the mind can conceive it. Repeat the mantra "*hamsah*" or "*hong-sa*" 16 times.

This practice is not for people who are not living clean, ethical, and spiritually focused lives. I am including it here as an example of how the techniques of yoga may blend together to bring the practitioner to deeper and deeper states. *Nadi Shodhanam* (described above) is a good preliminary practice, as are the *yama* and *niyama*.

Above I mention the idea that a person who practices yoga and wishes to experience palpable gains should have as a basis a spiritually focused life. These days a spiritual lifestyle with regard to yoga may seem untoward and old fashioned. A healthy, peaceful, stable lifestyle focused on virtue may not be in vogue or get someone media fame and fortune. It will, however, provide the foundation for the difficult and lengthy journey home to one's center of being. As Joseph Campbell claims in the opening of *The Power of Myth*,

We have not even to risk the adventure alone, for the heroes of all time have gone before us— the labyrinth is thoroughly known. We have only to follow the thread of the hero path, and where we had thought to find an abomination, we shall find a god; where we had thought to slay another, we shall slay ourselves; where we had thought to travel outward, we shall come to the center of our own existence. And where we had thought to be alone, we shall be with all the world. (cited in Moyers, 1988, Para. 2)

Somatic Practices

CHAPTER 1

CHAPTER 2

CHAPTER 3

CHAPTER 4

CHAPTER 5

CHAPTER 6

CHAPTER 7

CHAPTER 9

CHAPTER 10

References

Ballentine, R. (1999) *Radical Healing: Integrating the World's Great Therapeutic Traditions to Create a New Transformative Medicine.* Harmony Books.

Bharati, S. J. (n.d.) "Schools of Tantra: Kaula, Mishra, & Samaya." SwamiJ. Accessed on 06/03/2023 at www.swamij.com/tantra.htm.

Campbell, J. J. (1973) *The Hero with A Thousand Faces.* Princeton University Press.

Chaitow, L. (1991) *Palpatory Literacy: The Complete Instruction Manual for the Hands on Therapist.* Thorsons Publishers.

Cohen, B. B. (2012) *Sensing, Feeling, and Action: The Experiential Anatomy of Body-Mind Centering®.* Wesleyan University Press.

Cohen, B. B. (2018) *Basic Neurocellular Patterns: Exploring Developmental Movement.* Birchfield Rose Publishers.

Cohen, B. B. (n.d.) "Embodied Anatomy and the Nervous System: Body Mind Centering." Accessed on 06/03/2023 at www.bodymindcentering.com/product/the-nervous-system.

Dana, D. (2018) *The Polyvagal Theory in Therapy: Engaging the Rhythm of Regulation.* W. W. Norton & Company.

Demers, C. (2022, September 25) Polyvagal Theory and the Mind (Powerpoint). SYMT. Accessed on 06/03/2023 at https://www.spandayoga.com/_files/ugd/fa907b_dceba54e72164cec95efb1477b089d87.pdf

Feuerstein, G. (2001, Oct/Nov) "Does Modern Yoga's Innovation Disrespect Traditional Yoga?" Yoga International. Accessed on 06/03/2023 at https://yogainternational.com/article/view/does-modern-yogas-innovation-disrespect-traditional-yoga.

Godman, D. (2023) "Renunciation." Accessed on 27/07/2023 at https://www.davidgodman.org/renunciation

Goodbread, J. H. (1987) *The Dreambody Toolkit.* Routledge & Kegan Paul.

Hanna, T. L. (n.d.) "What Is a Somatic Practice?" Movement Meets Life. Accessed on 06/03/2023 at www.movementmeetslife.com/en/posts/what-is-a-somatic-practice.

Hartley, L. (1995) *Wisdom of the Body Moving: An Introduction to Body-Mind Centering.* North Atlantic Books.

International Association of Yoga Therapists (IAYT) (n.d.) "History." Accessed on 06/03/2023 at www.iayt.org/page/LearnAbout.

Iyengar, B.K.S. (2005) *Light on Life: The Journey to Wholeness, Inner Peace and Ultimate Freedom.* Rodale.

Mindell, A. (2011) *Dreambody: The Body's Role in Healing the Self.* Deep Democracy Exchange.

Moyers, B. D. (1988, June 21) "Ep. 1: Joseph Campbell and the Power of Myth—'The Hero's Adventure.'" Accessed on 06/03/2023 at https://billmoyers.com/content/ep-1-joseph-campbell-and-the-power-of-myth-the-hero's-adventure-audio.

Netter, F. H. (2022) *Netter Atlas of Human Anatomy: Classic Regional Approach.* Elsevier.

Peabody Montessori (n.d.) "Special Education." Accessed on 06/03/2023 at https://sites.google.com/rpsb.us/peabody-montessori/faculty-staff/special-education.

Porges, S. W. (2011) *The Polyvagal Theory: Neurophysiological Foundations of Emotions, Attachment, Communication, and Self-Regulation.* W. W. Norton & Company.

Porges, S. W. (2017) *The Pocket Guide to the Polyvagal Theory: The Transformative Power of Feeling Safe.* W. W. Norton & Company.

Samuel, G. (2008) *The Origins of Yoga and Tantra: Indic Religions to the Thirteenth Century.* Cambridge University Press.

Satchidananda, S. (1978) *To Know Your Self: The Essential Teachings of Swami Satchidananda.* Doubleday & Co., Inc.

Schwartz, A. (2018, June 31) "Somatic Psychology and the Satisfaction Cycle: Dr. Arielle Schwartz." Accessed on 06/03/2023 at https://drarielleschwartz.com/somatic-psychology-satisfaction-cycle-dr-arielle-schwartz/#.Y3o3jS2B3fd.

Stone, R. J. & Stone, J. A. (1999) *Atlas of Skeletal Muscles.* William C. Brown.

Timms, M. (1994) *Beyond Prophecies and Predictions: Everyone's Guide to the Coming Changes.* Ballantine Books.

Todd, M. E. (2008) *The Thinking Body.* The Gestalt Journal Press.

Todd, M. E. (2018) *Hidden You: What You Are and What to Do about It.* Martino Fine Books.

Vogler, C. (2007) *The Writer's Journey: Mythic Structure for Writers.* Michael Wiese Productions.

Watts, A. W. (n.d.) "Alan W. Watts Quotes." Goodreads. Accessed on 06/03/2023 at www.goodreads.com/quotes/7564722-you-are-something-that-the-whole-universe-is-doing-in.